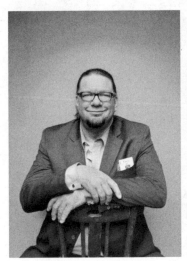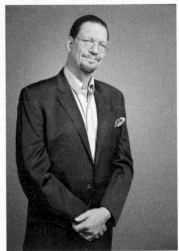

Before   After

PRESTO!

HOW I MADE OVER 100 POUNDS MAGICALLY
DISAPPEAR AND OTHER MAGICAL TALES

PENN JILLETTE

SIMON & SCHUSTER

NEW YORK   LONDON   TORONTO   SYDNEY   NEW DELHI

Simon & Schuster
1230 Avenue of the Americas
New York, NY 10020

First Simon & Schuster hardcover edition August 2016

SIMON & SCHUSTER and colophon are registered trademarks of Simon & Schuster, Inc. For information about special discounts for bulk purchases, please contact Simon & Schuster Special Sales at 1-866-506-1949 or business@simonandschuster.com.

The Simon & Schuster Speakers Bureau can bring authors to your live event. For more information or to book an event, contact the Simon & Schuster Speakers Bureau at 1-866-248-3049 or visit our website at www.simonspeakers.com.

Interior design by Ruth Lee-Mui

Manufactured in the United States of America

1   3   5   7   9   10   8   6   4   2

Library of Congress Cataloging-in-Publication Data is available.

ISBN 978-1-5011-4018-1
ISBN 978-1-5011-3953-6 (ebook)

Photo credits for page ii: Brad Trent (*before*); Frances George (*after*)

143.7

59.8

99.2

CONTENTS

SECTION THREE: EATING PIZZA IS VOTING FOR HILLARY 209

DISCLAIMER

You know the deal, right? There are legal requirements for anyone who writes anything about health to make sure he, she, or it is safe from lawsuits. Anyone can sue anyone, so you can never really be safe from a lawsuit, but you can make yourself less likely to suffer damage if a nut decides to file suit. When it comes to health, there's always a lot of jive about "see your doctor before making any changes in your lifestyle" and shit like that. And you skim over it like you do appliance warnings and Facebook privacy contracts, thinking, "Well, they have to say that, but it doesn't apply to me," and then you stick your knife in the toaster to get the bagel out and post a picture of the event to your social media without noticing your embarrassing reflection in the toaster. You figure that because you aren't a Darwin Award winner yet, you don't have to read disclaimers. You figure you already know the coffee at McDonald's is too hot to pour on your genitals—you don't have to read the cup.

This ain't like that. This disclaimer is not jive. This is a real, heartfelt, honest disclaimer. This was not written by lawyers—this was written by the guy who wrote this book. The guy who lost a hundred pounds. This is a disclaimer for the lawyers, but it also comes from my common sense, my concern, my knowledge, and my heart. This is a book about extreme personal lifestyle changes, written by a fucking juggler whose only higher education was Ringling Bros. and Barnum & Bailey Clown College. This book was written by someone who finished high school on a plea bargain. Someone who dropped his cock into a hot blow-dryer and scarred it like one of the Wendy's beef patties he no longer eats. This is a book written by an idiot. Take everything in this book with a grain of salt (but only a grain—salt is poison, as even this idiot now knows). I have *no* expertise. This book is about what I did, not about what you should do. Got it? This book is first-person, and you should not take it as second-person. Even I know a lot of what I did was wrong and stupid, but I don't even know which things were wrong and stupid. Even I, who dropped my fucking cock in a blow-dryer, knew enough to check with my doctor before making each change. If you're going to make any changes in your diet, exercise routine, or health, talk to your doctor—and take what even she says with a grain of nutritional yeast. Get a second opinion, and remember that my opinion does not count as the first opinion. I'm telling stories and making jokes. If you make lifestyle changes that you've checked out with your doctor, I hope this book can give you a few laughs, a little bit of moral support, and (I hope) some inspiration, but this is not a "how to" book. I'm okay with your thinking, "If that stupid fat fuck can do it, so can I." But I'm not okay with your doing what you think you understand that I think I understand I might have done that could have kind of gotten some results that might be good. Really, I don't know jack-fucking-shit! Okay? Be careful. Take care of yourself, and do not fucking trust me! Really. That's not legal jive, that's from my heart. It means a lot to me that you're reading this book, but please remember who wrote it: me.

If you take any lifestyle or medical advice from a juggler—you're an asshole!

INTRODUCTION:
HOW ARE YOU GOING TO DIE?

How do you think I'm going to die?

Most every night onstage, my partner, Teller, has a bullet signed and loaded into a gun by a stranger. He turns on the laser sight, aims the gun at my face, and pulls the trigger. *Bang!* The Bullet Catch is just a trick, but it's the most dangerous trick in show business. At least twelve magicians have died onstage pretending to catch a signed bullet. If you count carnies as magicians (and magicians don't), the number of people (if you count carnies as people, and many rubes don't) killed doing this trick jumps to over fourteen. These are men and women who were shot dead onstage in front of a live audience. When a magician fucks up a card trick, the crowd is simply more entertained than if the trick had gone as planned. When a magician fucks up with a gun and live ammo, the audience has nightmares for the rest of their lives.

Penn & Teller have done the Bullet Catch more than any other magicians in history, and it's a long history. The plot of this trick—sign the bullet, load the gun, shoot me—goes back to Native American magicians. I didn't even know there *were* Native American magicians before I worked on this trick. It doesn't seem like the wisest trick to use to entertain violent, invading foreigners. Our mentor, Johnny Thompson, had already lost two friends to the Bullet Catch when we started working on it, and he asked us to please not do it, but we felt we could do it safely, and Johnny knew we had a better chance of being safe with his help than without it, so he worked with us on it. Since we started doing the trick in 1996, I have had a gun fired at my face onstage 4,460 times. On any given night, chances are I'm staring down the barrel of a gun.

But the Bullet Catch will not kill me. Most likely, my death will not cause our audience members to be interviewed on CNN. I will die, like many Americans will, as a result of spending most of my life being a fat fuck. By the time I turned fifty-nine, I had been more than one hundred pounds overweight for over a decade. And before that I'd been fifty pounds overweight for over a decade, and before that I'd been thirty pounds overweight for over a decade, and before that . . . I was a homeless skinny teenager hitchhiking around the country who, for a brief, sexy statistical blip, might have been a little more likely to die from a gun than a doughnut.

No one has ever been seriously hurt working with Penn & Teller, and that includes Penn & Teller. We are tight-ass and careful. Safety in magic—safety in art—for me is more than self-preservation. Doing tricks in the safest way possible is more than just concern for my co-workers. Making dangerous-looking events safe is my job. That is the art. Letting dangerous things be really dangerous is not magic. That's not art. When we do tricks onstage that appear to be dangerous, we are asking the audience to enjoy themselves on our roller coaster. We want their visceral and their intellectual to collide at faster miles an hour. We're expecting them to feel their lizard heart race at the apparent danger while their human brain says, "It's just a show—they've never been hurt." In order for our art to be valid, in order for our tricks to celebrate life and health while thrilling the audience, those tricks must be safe. There are magicians who try to convince their audiences that the tricks really are dangerous. They try to convince the audience that their tricks aren't tricks. That's worse than lying. There are magicians who have been hurt, and there are more who perform cheesily staged "accidents" that are reported by a credulous, jaded media as real incompetence. The cynical business model is that the public will come to see their shitty acts in the hope that the show might contain real suffering and maybe death. This makes the audience complicit in unnecessary human risk. I don't know how many in the audience truly believe they are going to the theater to witness a clumsy, stupid, unskilled, careless asshole suffer and die, but if anyone really is, Penn & Teller don't want them in our audiences. We don't want them as fans. Fuck them in the neck. Shakespeare and *Call of Duty* are able to thrill people and celebrate life without anyone getting hurt. We want to be like them; we do not want to be like NASCAR.

The above paragraph is a self-righteous rant I've been spitting out for twenty years. I carry on about how precious life is and about how art, no matter how soaked in artificial blood and heart-racing terror, must always be safe. I show contempt for those of my peers who hang by their nipples from helicopters or pretend to come very close to drowning. And during the whole time I was preaching this, the whole time I was bragging about how careful we were and how much we loved life—I was closer to stroking out onstage from being a fat fuck than any of those assholes were to theatrical injury. And when I died, there wouldn't even be a good story. Roy of Siegfried & Roy gets his head bitten off onstage at the Mirage by a fucking tiger. How is that less artistic and beautiful than slo-mo death from fucking doughnuts?

It's not that simple, of course. Siegfried claims that Mantecore, the tiger, sensed Roy's high blood pressure and bit his fucking head off to save him. I believe that S&R believe that, but I don't believe it. If there were any chance of that being true, there would be more white tigers on the Mayo Clinic's payroll. If tigers could smell hypertension and wanted to fix it with carotid-artery bloodletting, they would have spent every performance biting more necks than Stefan Salvatore. People in Las Vegas are fat and dying because of it. Even if a bite to the neck would cure it, there aren't enough hungry tigers left in the world to save our fat asses.

I guess, statistically speaking, I will still die of some sort of heart thing. I was fat for a long time. It seems like age fifty-nine is a little too late to repent. But all the charts show that I have increased my life expectancy at least a bit by losing over a hundred pounds and eating better. I dismiss Roy Horn's medical-tiger treatment, but it sure isn't more stupid than me getting out of breath walking up a flight of stairs and not changing a goddamn thing. I ate a handful of pills every morning, I was in the hospital a couple of times a year—and I still ate like a pig. I ate worse than a pig—I ate like an American. Roy's assessment of Mantecore's motives is sage compared to my stupidity. Drowning while hanging by my tits from a helicopter while catching a bullet in my teeth is at least more exciting and life-affirming than feeling my vitality slide away because I'm in the habit of eating pizza.

Goddamn, I'm a fucking idiot.

Three months before my sixtieth birthday, I radically changed the way I ate. With the help of Ray Cronise—CrayRay, as I came to call him—I lost over a hundred pounds. I feel better than I can ever remember feeling. My doctors are all amazed. My family is no longer worried.

I didn't lose the weight in order to write a book. I didn't train myself to eat healthy in order to share my techniques with the world. I didn't do it because the trips to the hospital scared me skinny. I did it because I wanted to give myself a few more chances to die from the Bullet Catch.

SECTION ONE

JUST ANOTHER FAT FUCK

ONE-THIRD THE SIZE OF A COW DRESSED AS AN ELEPHANT

In 2014 I made a movie called *Director's Cut*. I wanted to play a bad guy. I wanted to be the psycho villain. I also wanted a villain who was an outsider. In the early drafts of the script, I named the character Herbert Khaury, which is Tiny Tim's real name. Tiny Tim is a hero of mine, but he was also an obsessive nut and a bit of a stalker. Maybe he was a bit more than a bit of a stalker. Maybe Tiny was a little dangerous. Tiny Tim had his problems. For the movie, I parted my hair like him and shaved my stupid beard. Tiny Tim didn't have a beard. Tiny was tall—not as tall as me, but still pretty tall, and Tiny was also pretty overweight by the time he was my age. So, being fat was good for the part. I was very happy being fat. At the time of that movie, I was the fattest I've ever been in my life. I thought fat was good for the part.

If you're reading or listening to this book right when *Director's Cut* comes out, you might see me on some talk shows pimping this book or read an interview or two with me. If you do, you'll hear me talk about gaining all that weight to play my character, Herbie, in the film. You'll hear me spin how fat I was. I don't like the word "spin." I prefer the word "lie." I'm going to be implying very strongly (lying) that I gained all that weight to play my character. It's the worst kind of lie, because by the time I'm done with it, I'll believe it. There will be some truth in it, so I can focus on that little truth until the big truth goes away. The weight sincerely was great for the character, and it really made everything perfect for that movie, but I hadn't spent thirty years getting fat because I was planning to play Herbie. I wrote the script about ten years before we shot it . . . but I can't produce any notes that are time-stamped from those days saying, "I sure better start eating like a pig to do my best acting." Maybe De Niro just got a hankering for spaghetti while working on *Raging Bull* and then just spun the press accordingly.

By the time you read this, I will believe that I gained over a hundred pounds for my movie; that in order to gain weight for my art, my sacrifice to the muses was to eat everything I saw. I know what it feels like to start spinning, progress to lying, and eventually believe the lies so much that you don't even remember that they started as lies.

In 2012 I went on *The Celebrity Apprentice* with Donald Trump, who has hair that looks like cotton candy made of piss. Before the show was over I published my previous book, *Every Day Is an Atheist Holiday!*, which stated that Donny's hair looked like cotton candy made of piss. I created the most perfect description of Donald Trump's hair ever given by anyone. "Hair like cotton candy made of piss" is also the phrase that Trumpy said was his reason for my coming in second a year later on *All-Star Celebrity Apprentice*. I love that about Trump. He comes out and admits crazy shit like that. He doesn't pretend he's not being arbitrary and petty. His charm is arbitrary and petty. It's supposed to be my job, as bitter loser, to claim that his real reasons were arbitrary and petty, but Trump fucked me on that. He's enough of a real, inspired nut that he just says outright what I would have to claim, and after he does that, all I can do is lie more and write that it was just that one joke, which it wasn't. Trump is the hero here, and I'm the bitter loser liar. He just made it easy for me.

Part of the final challenge was coming up with an ice cream flavor. If Trump had said that my competitor's ice cream really was better, which it wasn't, I'd have a beef; but nope, he was straightforward and honest, and I'm the weasel. My hair doesn't look like cotton candy made of piss, but it does look like the tail of a pathetic, aging roadkill raccoon. And if you said that to me, I wouldn't let you win a game I was running even if your ice cream made me cum, but I wouldn't cop to the real reason like Trump did. Trump was a better man than I . . . in this one very specific instance, on his show, with me, on that exact day. I'm as aware as everyone else that, since that one day with me, there is ample evidence that in general he is at very best the worst person who ever lived, and the best thing about him is that his hair looks like cotton candy made of piss. Believe me, I'm as horrified as you are. My ice cream was better, and my marketing was more successful, but I can be rude, weird, and crazy (and I guess I was), so I shouldn't have won. That's fair, but if I'm going to spin that fat ain't my fault, why not lie and say that Donald Trump's temporary, accidentally brave honesty is petty and arbitrary? I'm on a roll, spinning down a hill with my old-dead-raccoon-tail hair blowing in the wind.

Because of my arbitrary and petty rudeness to Mr. Trump, the people with intellectual disabilities at Opportunity Village, the charity I played Trump's game for, didn't get the quarter-of-a-million-buck first prize. But, thanks to Trump's honesty and my dishonesty, others involved with *The Celebrity Apprentice* wrote checks that actually totaled more than two hundred fifty grand. Exposure on Trump's show sold a metric shit-ton of tickets to *The Penn & Teller Show* at the Penn & Teller Theater in Las Vegas. So, I'm a bitter loser who won big by being rude and lying just a little bit. I'm actually the big *fat* bitter loser, because, you know, I gained all that weight to play the part of Herbie in my movie. I'm a real artist—a bullshit artist. I lie like a rug.

The ice cream I created, Vanilla/Chocolate Magic Swirtle, is still available at some Walgreens locations, but it'll probably be gone by the time this book comes out; as I remember, though, it's really good. I added sea salt (which is just salt) to dark chocolate, swirled that into vanilla ice cream, and threw in some caramel "turtle-like" candies. It's good ice cream. La Toya Jackson helped with the great name, and Dennis Rodman let me borrow his palate to get the vanilla base to just the right level of sweet and rich. It tastes great. It's sweet, rich, and comforting. I'd have an argument with my wife and then eat a whole container, and that's the grown-up way to live. It's really good ice cream, and you should try it if you ever get a chance. My share of the money goes to Opportunity Village, and it'll be your favorite food ever. And then you'll read the rest of this book and you'll never eat it again. I giveth, and I taketh the fuck away.

I take my acting fat seriously. Before the script was really finished, I changed my character's name from Herbert Khaury (it's not right to use Tiny Tim's real name) to Herbert Blount—Blount being jazz great Sun Ra's real last name. Sun Ra, another crazy hero of mine, was also really fat. Sun Ra was also from Saturn, so he had an even better excuse than gaining weight for a movie. As part of my dedication to the craft of acting, I'd have big fat steaks at the Musso & Frank Grill in Hollywood. I'd have big fat steaks everywhere. I ate a shit-ton of bread and butter and buttered popcorn and candy. And grilled cheese. And grilled cheese with bacon. And pizza. And pizza with bacon. I'd eat dozens of raspberry-filled Krispy Kreme doughnuts, which, I either read somewhere unreliable or made up, were Elvis's favorite dough-nuts. Yum. And Krispy Kreme doughnuts with bacon. Yup. For the past several years, I've hosted Penn Jillette's Private Bacon and Dough-nut Party, a private party coincident in time but not associated with James Randi's The Amaz!ng Meeting for skeptic and atheist cats and kitties in Vegas. I'd give everyone free bacon and doughnuts and play dirty-ass rock 'n' roll with nearly naked men and women all around me. It's all part of my plan:

> Sell ice cream.
> Give away bacon and doughnuts.
> Get really fat for a movie.
> Write this book to inspire all the fat fucks I helped encourage to get that fat.

I am Wile E. Coyote, Super Genius.

By the time we were done shooting *Director's Cut*, I was fat, depressed, tired all the time, and couldn't walk up a flight of stairs without panting. That's what a serious actor I am. At the end of every *Penn & Teller Show*, I run up the aisle to the back of the theater and into the lobby to meet audience members, sign auto-graphs, and pose for pictures, and will do so for as long as I'm still lucky enough to have people who want those things from me. At my fattest, at my Herbie movie weight, I couldn't do a very light jog *down* the five stairs from the front of the stage to the aisle without being winded. Even talking in the show was a bit of a strain. Yup—I'd get winded talking, and all I know how to do is talk. What the fuck? I don't know exactly what I weighed, because when I got that fat, I didn't really weigh myself much. But I was definitely north of 320 pounds. Truth be told, I probably hit 330. If I'm willing to beef up my accomplishments, let's spin that with a little goose and make it 333⅓, a little more than half the number of the beast and one-sixth of a ton. Yeah, I like that. One-sixth of a ton. Just six of me would make a ton. Wow, that's one-twenty-seventh of a shit-ton. Shit.

Around this time, we started using a live cow in the *Penn & Teller Show* in Vegas. A cow isn't a very glamorous animal for the Vegas Strip, so we dress her in elephant drag and call her an elephant. We think that's funny. An American cow with a feedbag trunk to make her look like an elephant—will that be viewed by future social critics in the same way we now view blackface? I don't know. I plan to be dead by then. The "elephant" in our show is the size of a small cow. A small cow that we call Elsie onstage. The two cows that play the part of Elsie are actually named Gecky and Star. We had nothing to do with those names, and I have no idea how much weight they each gained for the part. Gecky weighs 1,117 pounds. That's small for an elephant, and even a little small for a cow, but when the Vanish of Elsie, the African Spotted Pygmy Elephant went into the *Penn & Teller Show*, Penn weighed about one-third of her fake-elephant/real-cow weight. I was a third the size of a cow dressed as an elephant. I was a fat fuck. I was that fat because I take my acting craft seriously, and I like bacon.

I couldn't run or really talk, and I had hypertension that was supernatural. I used to walk around knocking on two hundred for the top number (I never notice the bottom number; who cares?). My permissive doc had me on massive doses of six different blood pressure drugs. I got up in the morning and took drugs that made me piss so much and so fast that I couldn't take them before I had to ride to the airport. I had to take them *at* the airport, because it's more convenient to piss five times on a flight from Vegas to L.A. than to pull the car over during the fifteen-minute ride to the airport.

Why did I have such bad hypertension? Because I was one-third the size of a cow dressed as an elephant! But I didn't see it that way. I knew that was part of it, but I couldn't believe that was all of it. I figured I would have high blood pressure anyway. My mom and sister had it, and I have some African- and Aboriginal-American ancestry, and it's . . . you know, genetic. I was born a fat fuck like you were born gay. Jesus fucking Christ, I'm an idiot.

My doc would tell me to lose weight, and I knew he was right, but . . . I didn't see myself as fat. Or, rather, I saw myself as fat but didn't see fat as a problem. My job didn't depend on my weight one way or the other. When I got acting jobs, I either played myself or a fat guy just like me. Penn & Teller were never sold as attractive sex symbols; we didn't have the sex-symbol hand to play. My showbiz success was not tied to my weight. I was married and didn't have to worry about getting fucked. Some people didn't use "fucking fat" as the first two words to describe me because I'm also fucking tall. I'm six foot seven, so I'm a big guy. "Big guy" includes "fat," but it's not *just* fat. I carried my weight really well, except for the blood pressure that was on the verge of making me drop dead or stroke out every second of every day. I was fine. I was happy, except for the constant depression and being winded just thinking about running to play with my children. I was a miserable fat fuck with such a great job, a great family, and wonderful friends that I was theoretically and psychologically happy even at one-third the weight of a cow dressed like a fucking elephant.

Oh, the things I've done for art!

DISCO DOC AND ENGLISH VOLTAGE BLOOD PRESSURE

In October 2014, after we wrapped *Director's Cut*, I went in for my annual physical. My doc strapped on the sphygmomanometer (one of my favorite words) and, even on every drug known to man in elephant-sized doses, my blood pressure had me on the edge of stroke-out. Doc said I had to see my cardiologist (that's right, I already had a cardiologist) to find out whether there was something that could explain this high blood pressure. We were pretending to look for something that was causing my hypertension while not talking about the one-third of a fake elephant in the room wearing a blood pressure cuff that was straining its Velcro around his fat-fuck arm. It's so easy to lie to yourself.

So I headed to my cardiologist. He came into his office like he was about to go to a disco. He was fashionable, trim, and active, like a commercial for Viagra. Big smile and some sort of sexy Latin accent. He obviously didn't need BP medicine or Viagra. He drew my heart on a piece of paper to show me constricted blood flow and shit like that. "Bro, you need to take off some weight, my man." I don't think he really said that, but he should have.

After he accurately diagnosed that my blood pressure was higher than Screamin' Steve Hawking's intelligence quotient because I was fat, he then joined me in pretending that diet wasn't the reason. Ignoring the sagging and groaning of the metal examination table beneath me, he said he had a test he wanted to run. Maybe I had some sort of blockage in my heart. If a guy comes into a doctor's office with a Hi-C can rammed up his ass, I guess the first thing you do is take a blood test to make sure the discomfort isn't due to a prostate problem. So I needed a test. In about a week, when I had a night off, I would go to the hospital. Disco doc would have his nurses shave around my cock, and he'd stick a needle into my groin with a camera on it and thread it up through my heart to have a look-see. This was an outpatient thang. It would take a couple of hours, and I'd be fine.

I wouldn't be unconscious for the groin threading, but they would give me a drug to calm me down and make me forget the pain. I think David Bowie took a drug like that and forgot the '70s. I didn't need to calm down—I wasn't nervous—but the idea of making someone forget the pain creeped me out. Dr. Daniel Kahneman, big fancy-ass Nobel guy, explains that he imagines us as having an experiencing self and a remembering self. The experiencing self gets all the pleasure and the pain in real time, and the remembering self makes all the decisions. So whether you get fucked in a good way or a bad way, it's the experiencing self that will feel it and the remembering self that decides whether you do it again. Doctors know that only the remembering self is able to sue, so their strategy is to fuck the experiencing guy and play to the remembering one. That's just *Black Mirror* creepy.

On the day, I went to the hospital and filled out all the paperwork. The nurses shaved around my groin and then put a hand towel over my cock so I wouldn't be embarrassed. I told them they could suck it and I wouldn't be embarrassed. Experiencing Penn and Remembering Penn were both fine with that, even before the drug kicked in. As the drug kicked in, the nurses asked what music I wanted. I said "Dylan," and just as "I Don't Believe You" finished up on the OR Spotify, Disco Doc—sure that my drugs had kicked in—changed it to hip-hop and was rapping along with it while he was snaking a needle through my groin to try to find some Charlie blockage in my Heart of Darkness.

He didn't miss a rhyme as he found a 90 percent blockage in my heart. A serious blockage, in the area called the "widow maker." It was really dangerous. Hard-core dangerous. Since he was right there in my heart, kind of as I was having a heart attack, he put in a stent and opened up the blockage. My heart was instantly better. I was fixed up. It wasn't quite outpatient anymore, but I would just stay overnight and be fine to do the P&T show the next night. I had no problems: hip-hop, high, and a towel on my cock—that's the name of my new album.

Perfect; my heart used to be blocked and now it wasn't, so my blood pressure came right down to normal, right? NO! I was one-third the size of a fucking cow dressed as an elephant! Getting rid of the blockage didn't seem to help my blood pressure at all. Weirdly, my BP was through the roof even after the blockage was opened up. They couldn't get my top number below, like, 220. Holy fuck, my systolic number was UK house voltage. I could charge my electric car on 220 in four hours. Two twenty is knocking on dead. My wife, EZ, was freaking. My manager, Glenn, started worrying about his house payments. I was too fucked-up to know anything. Experiencing Penn was in serious pain, and Remembering Penn was in denial. There are two unreliable narrators writing this. I don't know what happened.

Hypertension is the "silent killer"; it has no symptoms. Or, rather, it's not supposed to. But when you get up to UK voltage, where I've spent a lot of time, it's like having bees living inside your head. I could see my BP and feel it all over. Maybe all of this was psychosomatic. I don't know. I'm the last one to judge that, but it wasn't a great night.

Everything about that hospital visit kind of blurs over. They did some sort of blood test and figured that maybe the stent had fallen out or collapsed or whatever bad stents do. Experiencing Penn didn't have a vote, and Remembering Penn just remembered the hip-hop, the drugs, and the nice hand towel on my junk, so I was happy to have them snake the camera up the other leg and check out the stent.

All during this procedure, I still intended to do the show the next night. I'd never missed a P&T show. Never. If you want to play Broadway and have a bunch of millions of dollars invested in a show without understudies, your people must be able to say, "They've never missed a show." When I had pneumonia a couple of years ago (also not helped by my shitty diet and being a fat fuck), I would pull two IVs out of my arm every evening at six, go do the show, come back to the hospital, have the IVs replaced, and wait for my morphine. That was a bitch for both Experiencing Penn and Remembering Penn. We all remember that. I was nearly considering shooting up between my toes. It was miserable, but I didn't miss any shows.

Now I was arguing about how I was going to make the show that Glenn had already quietly canceled. When we went back to Broadway eight months later, you'd think the ads had to say, "They've missed only one show!" But they didn't say that. They said, "They've never missed a show." None of the investors or publicity agents are going to read this book or check Vegas hospital records, so fuck 'em.

They kept me in the hospital for a few days. The people who loved me were scared, but I didn't care. It just didn't seem like a big deal. I'd had blood pressure that high many times before, and I'd had blood pressure barely below that all the time. I had my CPAP machine (continuous positive airway pressure machine, which I had because I was too much of a fat fuck to even sleep without medical assistance), and they gave me drugs to make sure both ExPenn and RemPenn were doing fine. Nope, it really wasn't a big deal at all until the doc walked in and hit me with the news. He'd finally discovered the problem.

I was one-third the size of a cow dressed as an elephant.

OFFICIAL PERMISSION
TO GO CRAZY

The doc had discovered the problem, but it was EZ who first mentioned his solution to me. She said the doc was going to prescribe a gastric sleeve, an operation to shrink my stomach so it would be physically impossible for me to eat like a fucking pig. I would only be able to eat like a fucking medical research pig with a reshaped stomach. EZ and I didn't know much about stomach sleeves. We still don't, but in our limited experience, they work. EZ and I are good friends of Lisa Lampanelli's. She's a great comic. I was proud to have her in my movie *The Aristocrats*, and later she and I were on *The Celebrity Apprentice* together. For all the time I knew her, Lisa was a bit fat. She didn't need to be fat or to fuck African American guys in order to be funny, but for most of her career she was fat and fucking African American guys, so she talked about those things in her act. If you don't live it, it won't come out the horn.

She got some sort of stomach operation, and then suddenly she was thin. Not just thin*ner*, but thin. Skinny. She was thrilled about it. She was never funny because she was fat, she was funny in spite of being fat, and after the operation she was healthier, happier, and just as funny. It made sense to me that Lisa got the operation. She was fat. But it seemed odd that EZ was recommending I get the same operation. Well, it seemed odd to me. It didn't seem odd to anyone else, because everyone else knew I was fat. And because I said I was fat all the time, and called myself a fat fuck all the time, everyone assumed I knew I was fat. But I didn't *really* know I was fat. I thought I was big. A big guy. I had made peace with being a big guy. I didn't think 322 pounds was that bad for six feet seven inches. I carried all that weight really well. I'm a big, loud guy, and I was loud enough to carry a little more big. I claimed to be the rock 'n' roll animal. I was a big, loud comedy magician. I could shrug off my wife's stomach band suggestion. Let Lisa get all trim and thin—I was fine as a big guy. We just had to find the right drugs to fix a fellow who was clearly just genetically predisposed to hypertension . . . and about one-third the size of a fucking cow dressed as an elephant.

If I couldn't honestly see myself as really fat, I couldn't get really thin. I used to smoke cigarettes. I was a smoker who never bought a pack of cigarettes. Never. I smoke in the show after I do my fire-eating bit. It's showbiz to light a cigarette off my tongue and smoke it. It's a good way to show the fire is real. The fire in fire eating is real. Fire eating is real. Fire eating is not a magic trick. Fire eating is a skill. There is no cheat. As we say in the carny, there's no "G" on the joint, no affis-gaffis. Fire eating is done by combining a working sense of physics and human physiology with a natural lack of common sense. "Know nothing, fear nothing" is what my mom said about me. Besides being a pretty good fire eater, I did some cigarette magic tricks. I learned to palm them and "tongue" them (just what you'd think—the same as tonguing an asshole, except the asshole is doing the tonguing). I smoked cigarettes to do tricks with them, and then to close my fire-eating bit. I smoked cigarettes for professional reasons. I also started smoking them when I was sitting around with coffee after a meal. This was back when you could smoke in public. I'd bum cigarettes from friends who smoked and enjoy a smoke with them after dinner. And then another one. And sure, why not a third? One of the greatest days of my life was watching the Velvet Underground rehearse for their reunion tour in the '90s. They were getting ready to play their first show together since the '60s. I couldn't believe I was in a New York City rehearsal studio with some of my biggest heroes. I was watching Sterling, John, Moe, and Lou put together a show that I would later see in Wembley Stadium in London. A show full of the music that changed my life. The music that helped me become who I am. During that rehearsal, Lou took a break and said, "Hey, Penn, let's have a Carlton and a Moussy." Moussys were nonalcoholic beer and Carltons were cigarettes that didn't have much cigarette in them. Lou was cleaning up. For Lou, these were big steps toward better health. Me . . . I was just smoking.

My closest old buddy, Robbie, who worked on our crew, smoked. I would bum cigarettes from Robbie and smoke with him. I'd even bum cigarettes from guys on our crew who weren't really friends, just accommodating coworkers. I told myself I was bonding with them, but they knew I was just smoking. I felt guilty for all the cigarettes I took from all the crew guys backstage and on our movie sets, but not guilty enough to buy my own. I was cleverer than that. I had the movie prop guys buy cartons of all the brands that the crew smoked and then give them to the smokers on the crew; then I would bum cigarettes from everyone with a clear conscience. I'm such an asshole. And I was a smoking asshole.

I was probably smoking more than a pack a day, but I couldn't quit because I wasn't a smoker. I never bought any cigarettes. I was coughing every morning and getting headaches if I didn't have my borrowed cigarettes all the time, but I wasn't a smoker. One day when I was talking to a friend, I said out of the blue, "I guess I'm a smoker." That was the day I quit. Once I said that, I was able to take action. I still take a few drags after the fire-eating bit, so that's 10 percent of a cigarette every two weeks. That's .12 packs a year. That's okay.

When the doctor walked into my room and said we had to consider stomach sleeve surgery, I understood for the first time that I was a fat person. Not a "big guy"—you know, kind of meaning tall, too. Not a "fat fuck," with a smile and a wink. Let's get rid of that word "fat." "Fat" is a cruel word, but that's not the worry in this context. It's also very colloquial. It's an everyday word. It can be used as a positive. You can search for "fat cocks" on the Internet, and the images are proud. If you spell it "phat," you can search for all sorts of pornography, and even fashion and bling will pop up. "Fats" Domino invented rock 'n' roll. Fats was a genius who was very, very short. I know the word "fat" has caused untold suffering, but it still wasn't bad enough for me. But a doctor suggesting surgery—that made me *obese*. Now I had to see myself as obese. Could I shrug that off? On any chart you want to look at—not just the bullshit Body Mass Index but any chart—even for my height, body type, activity level, and muscle mass, I was obese. That's a word you can't spin nice. There are no "Obese Burgers"—at least, they're not advertised that way.

I was medically obese, and that's the reason I was in the hospital. That simple sentence had never occurred to me before. We didn't have to talk about genetics. Anyone as fat as I was would be sick. I was obese, and my doctor was recommending surgery to deal with the obesity that was causing my sickness. My obesity was what put me in the hospital, away from the show I never missed and the children I always want to be with. The suggestion of surgery was crazy. How fucked-up do you have to be to have surgery suggested as an option for lifestyle change? As crazy as obese me.

Up until that instant—lying in a hospital bed with blood pressure that couldn't be controlled, my groin shaved and snaked, with a 90 percent blockage just having been pulled out of my Heart of Darkness—it had never occurred to me that my weight was a problem. My doctor knew surgery was necessary to get me healthy, and told me so. He didn't equivocate; he said it outright, but he also expected me to argue. I could tell he had all his obese ducks in a row to explain why I needed this, to overcome the reservations he knew I would have.

I said: "Sure. Okay." I didn't put up the slightest fight. I smiled and nodded. I was down with him and his bad surgery self. After disarming him by agreeing immediately, I added, "But we can't do it right now, right? I can't go into the hospital for this operation because I'm already in the hospital for a procedure now? I need time to get over this one before I start my next hospital adventure, right? I have to leave the hospital in order to come back?"

"Yeah, we'll need to wait."

"Yeah, well, let's plan to do this in about six months or so, okay?"

Since he was so ready to argue and had done all the prep work, he wasn't able to take yes for an answer right away. But he also sensed I was up to something. He dispatched some of his ducks. He explained that a stomach sleeve was different from old-fashioned stomach-stapling. He explained that the operation had a high rate of success and was not a big deal.

"So, we can do that in about six months?"

"Yeah, that seems about right."

"And in the meantime, if I just happen to lose the weight, we don't have to worry about the surgery, right? What would you want me down to?"

"You'd have to lose a lot. A real lot. You gotta get down to two hundred seventy pounds ASAP. So you'd have to take off about fifty pounds right away. But the sleeve might get you down to two thirty, and at two thirty we might be able to get you off the meds. It's possible that at two thirty all your medical problems would go away."

What the fucking fuck? What the fuck? What? All my medical problems would go away?! He had been telling me for over a decade to lose weight, but I didn't think he meant I *had* to lose weight. I don't know what I thought he meant; I guess I thought he meant it would be nice, that it would make his job a little easier. I don't think he'd ever said before that my medical problems were obesity problems. I know now that's what he meant, but I'd never understood it before. My obese self had never been able to see it. I had told myself I was a guy with high blood pressure who was fat. I didn't know I was a guy who had high blood pressure *because* he was *obese*. There's a big difference between fat making something worse and obesity causing it. How would losing weight make my genetics change? Oh, that's right, I had been lying to myself. Genetics schmenetics—I was gobbling pills, sleeping with a machine strapped to my face, and feeling like shit because I was obese. Being an obese fat fuck was my medical problem. Wow. It had taken me twenty years to understand. Now what was I going to do about it? In six months I'd get my stomach sleeved, whatever the fuck that meant. The doctor gave me a website to check out so I could understand the procedure. Fuck that.

I've visited friends in the hospital who make hospital-bed proclamations like: "I'm going to eat perfectly from now on, and I'm going to hire a trainer. I'll hire two trainers. I'll hire three in case one of them gets sick from training me so hard." Those promises are more bullshit than any New Year's resolutions. Deathbed confessions aren't to be trusted. I don't trust anything anyone says on New Year's, in the hospital, or within ten minutes of cumming. I certainly don't trust myself at those times, so better not to make any promises in the hospital. I wasn't going to claim to my doctor and my wife that I was going to start eating right and exercising. I had no desire to do right. I never have desire to do right. I suck at right.

The doc's stomach-sleeve prescription gave me what I needed. It gave me something I had never had regarding my health before. That recommendation, that command, gave me the power to go fucking crazy. The doctor gave me the same gift that Tiny Tim, Bob Dylan, Sun Ra, Patti Smith, Lou Reed, Frank Zappa, Marcel Duchamp, Debbie Harry, Al Goldstein, Lord Buckley, Herman Melville, Nicholson Baker, Abbie Hoffman, Charles Mingus, Ayn Rand, Crispin Glover, David Allan Coe, Terry Adams, Andy Kaufman, Allen Ginsberg, Jack Kerouac, Jad Fair, and the Residents had given me. My doctor had just given me not only the license but the mandate, the life-or-death imperative to be crazy. To burn, to rage, to dance beneath the diamond sky with one hand waving free. I never wanted showbiz, or my art, or even my life to be normal. I didn't want to be adult and fit in with everyone else. I wanted to be a fucking nut. I always pushed for that in my job and in stories with friends, but I never ate nutty. I ate normally. I ate like a twenty-first-century American. I was a regular old American obese fat fuck on a regular old American diet. As far from crazy as possible. I was a fucking situation comedy. Getting surgery for being obese was extreme, so I had six months to take it to any other extreme I wanted. It was time to turn my health to rock-'n'-roll-free-jazz-beat-poetry-outlaw-transgressive-comedy performance art, and that's something I can do.

Doing health like everyone else certainly hadn't worked for me. I was obese like everyone else. I had high blood pressure like everyone else. I was on my way to diabetes like everyone else. I had a perfect life like everyone else, and I was still depressed like everyone else. I'd promised myself I would eat a little better like everyone else, and then I ate movie popcorn and cupcakes and doughnuts like everyone else. But that didn't mean I had to die exactly like everyone else.

I had six months to find something crazier than going back to the hospital for surgery just to stop me from killing myself by eating like a pig.

I had been given official permission to go crazy, but I didn't know how I wanted to use that power. I needed everything to sink in. I needed to get lucky. The seeds were sown, but they needed a little while to germinate in the piles of health bullshit in my head. Meanwhile, I started my grown-up "lifestyle change." I went on my half-assed '60s "hate Whitey" diet: I stopped eating all sugar, white flour, white rice, white pasta, and potatoes. Leave all the white food for the Klan. Fuck Whitey. That was easy. I stopped red meat (so, I guess I also hated Aboriginal Americans and Europeans, and maybe lemons). I got my sushi with brown rice. I ate my spaghetti sauce over quinoa. I got rich bread with wood chips in it. I ate oatmeal and nuts. Goudeau and I started taking hour-long trike rides. Goudeau is my great friend. He's my cohost on *Penn's Sunday School* and he wrote with us on *Penn & Teller: Bullshit!* We're both jugglers and we both have families. I love Goudeau, and Goudeau was wicked fat. We put our fat asses on racing trikes and did about an hour of light riding around the park. When I didn't trike, I used the rowing machine for half an hour.

The weight began to drop off me. "If you want to lose a lot of weight, first gain a lot of weight." Those extra twenty pounds that I'd just put on—some of the weight that I'll be lying about putting on for the movie—came off really quickly. I started weighing myself seriously at about 313 and I was down to 304 in five weeks. That's not bad. That's two pounds a week. That's very grown-up and sensible. Six months at that rate and I'd be down another forty pounds. I'd hit 289 by the time I promised to get my stomach sleeve. I might be able to alibi that to the doc: "Hey, man, I've made a lifestyle change like a grown-up. I should be down to 270 in another twenty weeks; another five months and I'll be where you wanted me to be to correct the emergency that put me in the hospital. That's cool, right?"

I felt better, and the eating was easy. I ate chicken and fish and whole-wheat pasta, and the weight came off. I loved the trike rides with Goudeau; we'd laugh and joke and ride, ride, ride. I weighed myself and watched each half pound slowly melt away. I had made my lifestyle change, but I still had my blank check for crazy. My heart was looking for a quick check-cashing payday predatory loan-shark place to cash it.

I was sniffing for crazy.

ENTER CRAYRAY—FUCKING HIS BRAINS OUT AT THE SWING CLUB WHILE THE CELIBATE TITTER

We do our *Penn & Teller Show* in the Penn & Teller Theater at the Rio All-Suite Hotel and Casino in Las Vegas, Nevada, in the United States of America. It's such a cushy gig. We do one show a night, so it's ninety minutes' work, five days a week, plus half an hour to get dressed each night. Add the commute, and it's a twelve-and-a-half-hour workweek. Sweet. I'm sixty years old, so that's a good retirement workweek.

I've fucked my cushy deal by loving every second of my job. I added an hour of live bebop jazz before the magic show. I play up-right bass. I get in an hour before every show and join Mike Jones, our monster piano player, and we play preshow bebop while people are getting in their seats and examining the props on the stage. That's another hour added to every show, and then after the show I'll pose for pictures, sign anything (when I'm lucky I get to sign a breast or two—they often come in pairs), and talk about anything with anyone who was at the show and wants to talk to me. So that adds another hour. After that I sit in our backstage "Monkey Room" and visit with any personal guests or dignitaries who were at the show that night. So my ninety minutes a night becomes a full ham-and-egger workweek.

There is no commercial pressure to change a show in Vegas. It's like the audience is touring. That's the conventional wisdom in this convention town. The other Vegas entertainers perfect their show somewhere else: NYC, Montreal, or on the road, and then bring it to Vegas and coast until death. They play golf all day and then go into their well-written, well-rehearsed, killer shows every night to make some pocket change.

Teller and I don't do that. We work constantly on new stuff—not just new bits for the live show but movies, TV shows, books, radio shows, podcasts . . . We love to work. I've turned my cushy twelve-and-a-half-hour-a-week job into a really cushy seventy-hour-a-week job that makes me the luckiest person in the world—except for the hypertension, being obese, and my doctor promising to make my stomach into a sleeve.

I was over a month into my "sensible lifestyle change." I was down at least eighteen pounds and feeling pretty smug as I ate my broccoli, spinach, and big hunk of salmon in the Monkey Room after the show. I was doing everything right. I was being a smart, health-conscious grown-up, but always in the back of my mind I knew I had a doctor's note to go crazy. I was in a slo-mo emergency situation. I had some freedom in reserve.

Wednesday, November 26—the night before Thanksgiving—is the night our story really starts. I came backstage with my room-service tray full of grown-up healthy salmon food. Jonesy, our piano player, was in the big comfy chair he'd commandeered. Teller was eating his after-show snack. My buddy Lana, who owned the Montessori school my children used to attend, and her husband and some children were on a couch; they had come in to see the new bit. They'd just seen us make a cow dressed as an elephant vanish, and they were eager to compliment. On the other couch was our friend Ray Cronise and his daughter, who was home on a break from college.

I have a few friends whom I refer to with the honorific "crazy." There's "Crazy James," a cocktail piano player in Frisco. Crazy James can do anything: he can cook, he owned restaurants, he's a great piano player, both cocktail and avant-garde. When I lived in Frisco, he'd knock on my door at 5:00 a.m. because he was wandering around the city and wanted to chat. I'd wake up and talk to Crazy James anytime; I love him. He once called in a motorcycle gang to enforce a contract he had with an accountant to do his taxes. That's another story. That's Crazy James.

There's "Crazy Kramer," who is a musical genius. He kinda sorta invented music in the '90s. Half Japanese, Butthole Surfers, and Nirvana all smelled a bit of Kramer's spirit. He played bass with the Fugs and GG Allin. Crazy James and Crazy Kramer are two of my oldest friends, and I'd take a bullet for either of them.

Ray Cronise isn't a traditional artist, and I didn't know him nearly as well as the others who shared that first name. Ray is a scientist and an entrepreneur. Compared with James and Kramer, he doesn't look very crazy. (Compared with Kramer, Charlie Manson doesn't look very crazy.) Ray doesn't say stuff that's too weird. I don't know why I use that affectionate term for him—I don't have the right. I still don't even know him that well. And he never really earned it like the others did, but I wanted to call him something besides Ray. "Crazy Raymond" sounds stupid. I don't like "Crazy Ray." "Cronise" doesn't do anything. But shorten "crazy" to "Cray," like my daughter says "cray cray," use "Ray," that drop of golden sun, for the second "cray," and you've got "CrayRay." It rhymes! It rolls off the tongue—and soon CrayRay would control most everything that rolled across my tongue. I didn't know him well enough then, but something about him made me think there was some depth and beauty and passion there.

Tim Jenison had introduced me to CrayRay some years back. Tim has been my friend since the '80s. We made a movie in Texas about Tim's obsession with painting a Vermeer called *Tim's Vermeer*. I have no idea why Tim isn't "Crazy Tim." I guess because Crazy Penn didn't happen to like the sound of that. Tim is a genius. Tim is the best of us, and Tim knows great people.

I cultivated a relationship with Ray for very self-serving purposes. Tim hinted that Ray could get me weightless—not in the diet sense, in the free-fall sense. Ray worked at NASA and then struck out on his own to start a company that would make astronaut training in the "vomit comet" available to civilians. I've told the story about my being weightless a zillion times. If you've heard the story of me stripping naked and singing "Barbarella" while weightless, well, CrayRay made that happen. (There's something about Ray and weight.) When I vomited in my hair during that flight, I also vomited on CrayRay. If you've seen the video on YouTube of me naked and weightless and vomiting in my hair, CrayRay shot that video while my vomit was running up and down his arm (we were weightless). One of the biggest adventures of my life started backstage on that Wednesday night, and it was all because of CrayRay.

CrayRay doesn't really know how to read a room. My friends wanted to talk about the Penn & Teller show they'd just seen, and have Penn and/or Teller (preferably Teller) hold court and tell stories from the six years we spent working on making a cow dressed as an elephant disappear. They wanted to hear stories of hauling Elsie's cow-ass in a trailer across the Vegas Strip for her show every night. They wanted to feel showbiz. Ray was sitting next to his daughter on the couch with Teller. CrayRay didn't feel the post-show-mingle-with-the-stars vibe; he had good stories of his own, and he was taking the floor.

He was talking a blue streak. He was on a water fast—just water. Before that he'd been eating only potatoes. As an experiment, he'd gotten rid of his diabetes with diet and then got it back with diet, and then lost it again. He had a glucose monitor embedded in his skin. He had a backpack that he wore to measure his exact metabolism, and he wore it while climbing seventy-four flights of stairs. Did we know that climbing those stairs took the amount of energy you'd get from just 2.75 Oreo cookies? "I want to do for nutrition what Tim did for Vermeer. Nutrition is my painting, my art."

His daughter, Alexia Raye, didn't say a word; she just sat and listened to her dad. She looked healthy. CrayRay looked thin. A healthy thin, I guess, but thin. Did we know that if you gave yeast a low-calorie diet, it lived longer? A lot longer? Mice, too. "Exercise is bullshit." CrayRay underlined "bullshit" in his speech because he knew that was the name of our television show. He pushed himself to swear more than he normally does, because he knows that offstage I swear a lot. CrayRay explained that our lives are just one long meal interrupted by a little work and maybe a little fucking.

> "Seasons matter; we keep storing fat for a winter that never comes."
> "We live in perpetual summer, electric lights and warmth; we never get cold. We sleep in overly hot rooms and still use blankets. Cold showers can stop depression. We treat SAD with warmth and light, but cold and dark do better."
> "Wear a cold vest and eat only potatoes. Potatoes are just a 'fuck you' to the paleo people. They have some stuff right, but they're wrong about so much more."
> "You don't need animals to make fat for you; you can make your own."

CrayRay was on a roll. He didn't notice Jonesy rolling his eyes, or Lana and her family looking over at me and waiting for a joke. Real scientists don't even try to read the room. Why should they? Information doesn't care what room it's in, so why should they? But the room was telling me I had to say something; the room wanted it. The ability to read the room is the character fault of entertainers. I wanted to listen to CrayRay, but the room demanded I do some schtickala.

In my best smarmy talk-show-host fake-questioning asshole voice, I asked, "Just potatoes for two weeks?"

And CrayRay was off again. Potatoes are "white" and considered bad, but people can live on potatoes for a long time. Did we know how much protein was in a potato?

"Speaking for the group, we don't."

Now we were all making fun of goofy, skinny science boy. Even CrayRay could sense we were rolling our eyes a bit. He wasn't *completely* blind to the room, and he knew the stuff he was saying flew in the face of everything all the smart, not-crazy (and very fat) grown-up people in the room knew. We were all unhealthy from our diets, rolling our eyes at the healthy guy.

There's a swing club in Las Vegas called the Red Rooster. People go there and have sex. They fuck strangers, they fuck friends, they fuck their wives and husbands. They fuck in front of other people and in groups and sneak off into corners and private rooms. There's food there, and sometimes a live band. A good-looking young pickpocket I knew in Vegas told a bunch of us how he had gone to the Red Rooster. He said some of the people weren't that attractive, and that these assholes were just fucking each other everywhere, on couches and in corners, and there was fellatio and cunnilingus, and they were just flirting and then fucking right there in the room. These middle-aged losers were just fucking everyone in sight. The pickpocket was getting big laughs rolling his eyes and making fun of the "swingers," these people who weren't as attractive as he was who were having sex with each other, while he and his girlfriend were just sitting there laughing. I had a question for him: "So let me get this straight: these other people were meeting people, having sex, and having a blast, and you were fully clothed and giggling and not fucking—and *they* were the losers? That's what was happening?"

It was the same thing with CrayRay backstage. We all knew about nutrition. We knew that frequent meals, exercise, and lots of protein were the answer. Everything had to be done in moderation. You couldn't do fast weight loss like CrayRay was doing. You couldn't fast or just eat potatoes. If you lost weight like that, you got sick, and then put the weight right back on. It wasn't healthy.

Yup, CrayRay was fucking healthy, and we were fat and laughing at him.

JOINING THE CULT

The day after CrayRay's backstage rant was Thanksgiving. I started the morning with twenty minutes on the rowing machine: very grown-up. I played Go Fish with the children and picked up friends and relatives at the airport. Those were my Thanksgiving duties. I had been advertising the sous-vide cooking appliance company Sansaire on my podcast, and EZ cooked up the turkey with our own Sansaire unit. EZ, Moxie, Z, my mother-in-law, and a few invited friends all had a great supper. My buddy Matt Donnelly described the sous-vide turkey as "turkey-infused turkey." I didn't eat myself sick, but I did eat a bit of everything, and I was pretty full. It was a great meal, but everything CrayRay had said was still echoing through my head. I wrote and asked him about the diet: could he get me down to 270 or 260?

"Sure."

"You know the doctor said that at about two thirty, all my meds go away."

"Let's do that, then."

"How hard is this?"

"Easy. Wanna go to two twenty? Lower?"

I told him that my doc was pushing for a stomach sleeve. CrayRay wasn't that crazy. He didn't want me to even consider that. "Just lose the weight and make your diet healthy." You'd think that with me actively interested in his diet-shit obsession, CrayRay would be even more full-bore eager to push it, but that wasn't the case. He was always full-tilt, whether people cared or not, and the amount of interest he got back didn't change his style at all. That's one of the many things I love about him.

The stuff he was saying was batshit crazy. It was all stuff I'd always felt was true, but all the grown-ups told me wasn't true. He said there wouldn't be frequent meals to "keep the metabolism going," that you didn't lose weight by eating more. He said I wouldn't exercise while I was losing weight—I'd get to my target weight and *then* exercise. He said I could lose more weight sitting on the couch and not eating. It was crazy stuff, but nothing he said seemed crazier than getting fucking surgery to not be fat. I was getting sucked into CrayRay's world. I could feel it. I would never have considered it without my doctor's note, but I had that, so I just let myself be sucked into the cult. He could be my Charlie, and I would be his Squeaky.

But first I wanted to check in with Tim Jenison. Now, anyone who's seen *Tim's Vermeer* knows Tim is crazier than a shithouse rat. After his youngest daughter left for college, the empty nest got to him, so he learned Dutch, reinvented a machine that seventeenth-century Dutch master painter Johannes Vermeer might have used to paint, built an exact copy of Vermeer's studio, and spent years painting his own masterpiece with that machine. Tim is a nut. I knew CrayRay had been there, helping Tim build the Vermeer room. Tim is wicked smart, and Tim loves science. CrayRay is right there with him. Tim really cares about truth. CrayRay is right there with him. Tim likes to see things proven wrong, especially things he himself believes. Tim is a good man. Fucking crazy.

So I called Tim and asked him about Ray. Tim said he didn't really know anything about what Ray was up to now. He knew that at one time Ray had worked for "government NASA" (Tim is a real libertarian), but he liked CrayRay anyway. I told him I might turn control of my diet over to CrayRay. Tim said, "He's a good scientist." That's a little like John Coltrane saying, "He's a good musician." What more could I want?

Since then, I've learned a little more about CrayRay's background. He's not a doctor. Not an MD or a PhD. He's a Southern boy, calls himself a redneck, and lives in Alabama, but *Huntsville*, Alabama. As in NASA Alabama. When Tim Jenison first introduced me to Ray, Ray was working at NASA and trying to get ZERO-G off the ground. I guess Ray had been short-listed to be an astronaut. Tim said Ray also had other weird government stuff in his past. Stuff he doesn't talk about. *Saturday Night Live*'s Dana Carvey's brother, Brad, also had some sort of background like that. Brad is the person Dana's character Garth in the movie *Wayne's World* was based on. He also has government time he doesn't talk about. I don't even know what that means. Neither Brad nor Ray talks about their government time, and I don't ask. CrayRay and Brad might have been meter maids for all I know.

As a libertarian, I'm not thrilled with the idea that NASA exists. I think all space exploration should be private, but if you have to work for a government agency, it might as well be NASA. And CrayRay had worked for NASA.

He left NASA and got into the swimming-pool business. Is that what a government guy would do? I don't know. Is that part of the re-volving door for lobbyists? I don't know. There's something not quite right about CrayRay. He's my kind of guy. When he got me weightless on his private vomit comet, it was a little shady. Shady like a beat-up

Mexican cargo plane with me and Billy Gibbons from ZZ Top on the manifest as "advisors" or something. There seemed to be much too little paperwork for a plane that was going to fly vertically straight down toward the ocean while we floated around. But Billy and I were on board with CrayRay. Billy played his guitar, and I stripped naked and threw up on CrayRay. Rock 'n' roll.

I had trusted CrayRay with my life in the vomit comet, and Tim said he did good science, and that was good enough for me. I asked CrayRay what he'd do. He said he had a program that he'd take me through. He mentioned two weeks of potatoes, but I didn't figure that was for me. He said I'd lose a lot of weight and agreed with my doc that I would probably be able to get off my blood pressure meds. I said it wasn't all weight; some of it was genetic. He said that was bullshit; I would get off the meds. He said I would feel amazing. He asked for ninety days: twelve weeks. Those are two different things; twelve weeks is eighty-four days. What CrayRay wanted was a season. CrayRay cares a lot about seasons. He says everyone seems to be able to stay on any diet for one full season—three months, twelve weeks, ninety days (all different amounts of time, by the way).

I had always dreaded diets, but there was one part of them that was really exciting: the test part. The performance art. If you want to know everything you need to know about Penn & Teller, it all comes down to masturbation. Neither one of us was told about masturbation when we were children—not by parents, friends, or school. So we each thought we had discovered it. That tells you most of what you need to know about us. Teller and I like to feel that we've invented something. Teller will hold a card in the palm position in his hand and think it's a new magic move because he turns his body a little bit to one side. He "solves" how to sit in his car. I get ideas and write them down and spew them forth and think they're brand new. I feel that way only because of ignorance. Someone has always covered everything I've thought before, but I don't like to think about that.

Part of that is just being American. Real American exceptionalism is simply thinking we're exceptional. Teller and I did a show called *Penn & Teller's Magic and Mystery Tour* (man, I hate that title; I didn't invent it!). We went to Egypt, China, and India. We talked to magicians around the world. I guess I'm supposed to write that it amazed me how much we all had in common. But what really struck me was the big difference in the way in which we bragged. All of them—especially the Chinese magicians—bragged by not taking credit for anything. They would show us brilliant moves, and when we complimented them, they would say they had learned them from their master, and that he in turn had learned them from his master, that they were ancient Chinese magic traditions. It was clear they would have claimed that even if they were showing us a trick that involved an iPad. Part of what made them proud of their work was claiming they were simply continuing an ancient tradition. They did not seem to take any pride in anything personal they created. Whereas American magicians—or at least Penn & Teller—will take individual credit for anything we can get away with. If I could get away with the claim that I had invented playing cards, I would do that. "Oh, yeah, I think Teller inspired me on the diamonds, but I just thought of hearts, clubs, and spades myself—they just kind of popped into my head."

Teller and I both thought we had invented masturbation. That's the similarity. We both have inflated ideas of our creativity. That's the similarity between us. I don't know how many other people think they invented masturbation, but we are both so sure of our creativity that in each of our hearts we believe we invented even vital bodily functions. Our differences are also shown in our discovery of masturbation: when Teller had his first orgasm, he thought he had injured himself internally. That's all you need to know about him.

We know you know how Teller discovered masturbation—I just told you—but how do I know? Think of your coworkers. Do you know how each of them discovered masturbation? I know about Teller because back when we were carny trash (we still are, I guess, but I mean back when we performed in an actual tent and not in a hotel/casino), we drove around together all day every day, ate every meal together, and shared a room at Motel 6 every night. We spent years talking to each other. Some of that talk was pretentious, highfalutin bullshit that Teller and I believed then and still believe now with all our hearts. Some was magic and comedy theory. Some was arguing about minutiae; Teller and I can put too fine a point on anything. But some of that talk was just killing time, so we talked about how we discovered jacking off. Teller thought he'd injured himself and was going to die from loss of precious bodily fluids.

I, on the other hand, thought it was an endurance test. I was in the bathtub rubbing my penis. It was hard in both senses. And rubbing it felt really intense. I'd done it a few times before, but I wondered this time if I could really push myself, if I could go for the world record for penis rubbing. At that time I didn't know I had any competition. I was inventing it, and was the best at it. From the second time on, right up until now, it was pure pleasure, but that first time was just to see if I could do it. If I could do it a little longer than before. I love a challenge.

Losing weight as a grown-up is supposed to be no challenge at all. People do everything they can to make it easy, and that takes all the fun out of it. Then they just fail. There's no fun for me in making something easy. I learned to juggle the way I learned to masturbate—no, not by dropping my balls on the cellar floor, but by seeing how far I could push myself. I didn't want to learn a three-ball cascade just well enough to impress people at a party; I wanted to be able to juggle three balls for three hours without missing once. If I dropped a ball after two hours and forty-five minutes, I'd start again. When I learned to ride a unicycle, I wanted to ride it thirty miles uphill to the giant hippie Brotherhood of the Spirit commune (renamed the Renaissance Community in 1974) near my hometown to hear their band, Spirit in Flesh, play. I'd ride it to school in the middle of the winter after a big snowfall. When I learned a juggling trick right-handed, I then wanted to learn it again left-handed, even though no audience would ever care. This is the juggler state of mind.

Magicians are the opposite. Magicians are always trying to get away with shit. "Can I do this and fool people into thinking I'm doing that?" That's all magic is. Magicians always want to brag that they invented an easier way: "You know, you don't need to do that fancy move; you can just mark the cards." "You could just use a stooge for that." Making it easy, just getting by, is a matter of pride to a magician.

Here's magic "low-fat fat": if you use it, you can eat the same way and still lose weight. Or magic "fake sugar": with it, you can drink soda all day and still lose weight. Never mind that it doesn't work, and worse, that it's not fun. It's magical thinking in both senses—magical thinking in that it doesn't work, and in thinking like a magician to make it easy. Take something impossible and do it the easy way. Cheat and fail anyway. That's not thinking like a juggler discovering masturbation in the bathtub, that's a magician discovering masturbation and thinking he needs to go to the ER. Teller is a magician; he wants to make things easy. I'm a juggler; I want to make things hard, and not just my dick. Difficulty is pride to a juggler. Pride in difficulty made me discover masturbation and helped me lose a hundred pounds.

Let's talk about children. There's a thing called the Stanford Marshmallow Experiment. In the '60s and '70s a professor named Walter Mischel conducted experiments in delayed gratification with young children. He put them in a room with a treat, like a marshmallow, and told them that if they didn't eat that treat for fifteen minutes, they would get more treats—but if they ate that one, that was it; they wouldn't get any more.

Follow-up studies showed that the children who could delay gratification did better for the rest of their lives than those who wolfed down the treat. Okay; but I can't help thinking that the ones who just said fuck it and ate the marshmallow right away grew up sexiest. There were many techniques that those able to delay used. Some hid the marshmallows from themselves, some looked out the window, some got lost in play to pass the time and take away the temptation. Those techniques work, but they're the easy ways; there's a little magical thinking going on there. The test subjects who grabbed my imagination were the ones who just sat there staring at the tempting, forbidden treat for fifteen minutes. Just stared at it. Smelled it. Thought about it. How groovy and intense is that? Those are the subjects I want to watch through life. I never got to take the test, but that's how I'd like to see myself acting. Put that fucker on my nose and make me balance it there for fifteen minutes. Make me put my mouth around it but keep my mouth open. And go longer than fifteen minutes. Please let me prove it all night. That would bring me the most joy. I may be known as a Las Vegas magician, but I'm really a puritanical Massachusetts juggler.

CrayRay tapped my inner masturbating juggler. He knew that Kennedy said we chose to go to the moon not because it was easy but because it was hard, and recognized that I would lose a hundred pounds because it was difficult. I wanted to feel like I was *doing* something. I wouldn't hide food or look out the window, I would stare at the marshmallow for ninety days, or twelve weeks, or three months— and at the end of whatever the fuck amount of time it took I would get my treat, and my treat would be not fucking dying with a stomach sleeve. Delayed gratification done like a juggler.

Before CrayRay got his claws into my psyche, part of my sensible grown-up weight loss plan was taking hour-long trike rides most days with Michael Goudeau. While I was fooling myself that portion control could work and that fatty fish was a weight loss food, I also thought that exercise would help me lose weight, so I was riding the trike. In a later chapter we'll cover the idiocy of trying to outrun your mouth, the idea that exercise can negate eating. That's just insane. But I was exercising like a grown-up with my buddy Goudeau. Yeah, motherfucker, I put "grown-up" and "tricycle" in the same image.

We ride trikes. They're low to the ground, with two wheels up front and one in the back. When you're riding them, you feel so spiffy. You fly along so fast, so low, like race car driving or War singing "Low Rider." You're not up high on what trike riders call a "launcher," a traditional bike with a racing seat that cuts off all circulation to your cock and balls. You're flying along in an easy chair. When you take a rest, you can stay right in your seat. You can ride a trike without making your cock go numb. You can ride right up and have sex without having to dance around to get the blood back in there. When you're riding a trike you feel so cool, but to everyone else you look like an asshole.

Riding a trike is like being Don Johnson: feeling cool while everyone knows you're a dipshit. I kind of enjoy that. I did the opening show of the second season of *Miami Vice*, and I sure didn't like a moment of being around Don Johnson, but it seemed like it might be okay to be Don Johnson. Yeah, I thought he was a dipshit, but he seemed to think he was pretty cool. Better than the other way around, right?

So, Goudeau and I are riding around the bike path near his house on our trikes and we're feeling like Don Johnson. We're feeling like a pair of wicked-fat Don Johnsons. I'm about three weeks out of the hospital at this point, and I'm dropping weight in a grown-up way.

I'm still on track to have a stomach sleeve, but I'm making some progress.

Goudeau is friends with CrayRay, too, and they had been talking about some of his crazy cold and diet stuff. I told Goudeau that I had gotten in touch with Ray and was maybe going to try his crazy thing. Goudeau said he was on board. Goudeau wanted to do it with me. I was surprised he came on board. Goudeau likes to cook, and really likes to eat. Goudeau is a coon-ass from Louisiana, and he likes his salt and fat. But he was also sick of being sick and fat.

When I told CrayRay that Goudeau and I wanted to do it together, he was against it. He didn't want me to talk to anyone about what I'd be doing, not even while I was doing it. He said that if Goudeau and I were doing it together, we would talk to each other and find ways to undermine it. He said it was like Fight Club, that we couldn't talk about it. He didn't want us talking to anyone. The first rule of CrayRay is don't talk about CrayRay.

I talk about everything I do. If you've read my books, or if you're reading this one, you know that. I'll talk about Teller discovering masturbation. I'll talk about herpes. I don't care. I like to share ideas. And now CrayRay was telling me his rules said that I couldn't talk to anyone about this. That's the moment I knew I'd be joining a cult.

One of the first things a cult does is cut you off from your family and friends and make you submit to a charismatic leader who you need to believe has all the answers, even if he goes against the beliefs of everyone else you know. CrayRay was going to cut me off from everyone, put me under a great deal of stress, and contradict everything I knew to be true. He was going to limit my ability to judge anything he was telling me. He was going to make me feel alone and go to only him for friendship and guidance. He was going to take control of my life.

I told him he was doing cult shit, and he said, "Yes."

How the fuck do you argue with that? My doctor had told me that I was going to get a stomach sleeve. They were going to cut into my body and change my digestion forever. How much worse is joining a cult? It couldn't be that much worse.

Okay.

So I signed up.

Goudeau and I told CrayRay that we would join his cult and do everything he said, that we wouldn't question it even between the two of us, and that we wouldn't talk to anyone else. We kind of hoped he wouldn't tell us the Beatles wanted us to kill the president . . . but we were in his hands.

When he'd talked backstage about two weeks of eating nothing but potatoes, I figured that was some nutty experiment that he'd done on himself or on college students or something. I didn't think I'd be eating nothing but potatoes. Also, as the brilliant magician Mac King once said about me, "You exaggerate way more than anyone else in the world." I figured that other people exaggerate, too, so "just potatoes" didn't mean *just* potatoes. It meant something else.

I didn't know what it *did* mean, but it sure didn't mean we were going to eat nothing but potatoes for two weeks.

Helter Skelter.

MAYBE I'VE EATEN ENOUGH GREAT FOOD

CrayRay said to me, "Maybe you've had enough great food." I had no idea what he was talking about when he said it, but now I get it.

Everything in this book should be taken with a grain of nutritional yeast, because we don't know how I'll end up. By 2017 I may weigh four hundred pounds and claim I'm working on another movie. I might slip back badly. I might fall off the unsalted hay wagon, but for right now, it feels great. And it's really easy.

That seems to be a recurring pattern with me: the stuff that's supposed to be hard is easy, and I get fucked-up by the easy stuff. There was a great British TV show called *Cracker* that starred Robbie Coltrane, who is an amazing actor and, with *Cracker*, had the perfect show for his talents. Someone had the stupid idea of bringing it to the USA in the '90s, and the even stupider idea of considering me to play his role. I guess they thought the fact that Robbie was a big guy was more important than his stunning talent, so they had me audition.

I don't mind auditioning. I go in with the attitude that I'm going to fail, so I might as well have fun. I often tell the person running the audition that if they want the character to be exactly like me, then I'm their man. Sometimes they want that and get me. But sometimes I do performance art at my auditions. "Performance art" really means I act like an asshole. I went up for a part in *Wall Street* and read for Oliver Stone the day after he won the Academy Award for *Platoon*. In the waiting room was every great actor in New York City, and they were all dressed wicked Wall Street-y. I was wearing a leather motorcycle jacket and some sort of hat advertising a tractor company. I was unshaven and wearing dirty sneakers. I probably looked like a twenty-first-century billionaire, but I was auditioning in the twentieth century. They were running behind, and I was waiting in the appropriately named waiting room. I had a show that night on Broadway, so I was going to have to split without auditioning if they made me wait much longer. They got to me right at the eleventh hour, and I went in. I guess Oliver Stone is a genius. People love his movies. He's very intense. Probably a genius. But, we kinda didn't hit it off. The moment we saw each other . . . well, the moment I saw him, I was uncomfortable. He commented on me looking like shit at an audition for *Wall Street*, and I said I thought he was a genius and could use his imagination to shave me and put me in a suit. I think the record shows that I'm already the asshole in this story. Can we call it performance art?

I knew I wasn't getting the part, so there was nothing riding on the audition. If I succeed in an audition and get the part—that's the story. If I'm not going to get the part, then I need to manufacture an interesting loser story. It was clear I wasn't getting the part, so it became time to make a story out of it. There was a poster up behind Mr. Stone for *Platoon*—don't forget, it had won the Oscar the night before! I said, "You know what you should have done with *Platoon*?"

"What?"

"I have an idea for your movie."

"What are you talking about?"

"You should do *Platoon* just the way you did it, but then, when it goes to credits, you should have outtakes, like in *Cannonball Run* or Jackie Chan movies. Have, like, a take of Charlie Sheen with the leech on his face saying, 'Does this look like a fucking anchovy or something?' And, 'Isn't that gook supposed to fall down when I shoot him?' Stuff like that."

I was getting my story. Oliver Stone said, "That would have ruined the picture." He wasn't clueless; he was fucking with me back. But all I wanted was a story . . . so I'm fine with part of the story being me getting fucked with.

"Well, maybe for your friends it would ruin it, but for my friends, it would have shown that you know you're just making a fucking Hollywood movie, and even though the subject matter is serious, it's still just a jive-ass way to sell popcorn."

He wasn't buying it and was growing bored with fucking with me.

I said one more hard-core asshole thing like, "Well, let's not argue about it, just pull back half the copies and put my ending on, put them back out, and see what the people think. You're a man of the people."

I had my story. Now, the temptation in telling this story is to make it look like I was brave and Oliver was an asshole. Nope. The truth is that Oliver does everything right in this story, and I'm the asshole. I'm an asshole. Especially when I'm going for a story. It's performance art.

He turned to the casting director and said something like "Can you imagine putting this asshole in a movie?" The casting people tried to explain that other people had done that, maybe because I had a show. He let me audition for the part (see? I told you he was the hero in this story). I was awful, and he told me so. I agreed. I had my story, and it was time to leave, but he had another idea. He said, "Let's have him read for a different part."

He gave me the part of an asshole to read. He asked me to take it out to the other room and work on it. I said that I had a show and didn't have time, but I'd read it cold for him if he wanted. I read cold for him, and that was that. I wasn't good at that role, either. As I left the room, I said to all the other actors waiting to audition, "Be careful—Oliver is going to talk to you about his personal relationship with Jesus." There was no reason to say that—I already had my story—but I thought it was funny.

I think it was Mariel Hemingway who leaned in the door and said, "I've met him before, Mr. Stone, and he's crazy." She had, and I am.

But there are two more punch lines coming:

I got the part! When my agent called and told me, I told her they made a mistake and they wanted Teller (he had auditioned straight and not gone for the story). I told her to call them back and tell them they just had the name wrong. My agent did that, but, damn, Oliver did want the big asshole.

So I shot *Wall Street* and worked with Oliver Stone and Charlie Sheen, and it was a one-day shoot for me and a nutty set. Charlie liked me, and we got along great. What more do you need to know?

And then a couple of months later I was in a trendy NYC restaurant hobnobbing with my fellow wizards. There were showfolk all around. Oliver Stone came over to my table, hardly leaned in at all, and said, loudly enough for everyone around to hear, "Hey, Penn, we just couldn't find a way to make your scene work in the new picture, so you're cut out." And there we go. Oliver Stone wins every showbiz round.

But I got a good story.

When I went to audition for *Cracker*, I went in knowing I wasn't a good actor. That gives a fellow a lot of power. As Neil Young sang, "It's hard enough losing without the confusion of knowing I tried." I don't have that confusion. I've never worked on acting. I'm a performer, not an actor, and that allows me to suck and not feel bad about it. I had the balls to audition with Robert De Niro and I acted with Michael Keaton, and because I never set out to be an actor, I'm okay sucking even in company that underlines that sucking. If you know you can't play basketball, playing with Michael Jordan would just be fun, right? It takes all the ego out.

Somehow I got through the first audition and got a callback. And all of a sudden it seemed like I might have a chance at starring in the American version of a brilliant British TV show, and I started caring. I went to see my friend the brilliant actor Dean Cameron (I call him Dino), and he worked with me. He also worked with me when I acted the part of a death row inmate in the Off-Broadway play *Exonerated* with Mia Farrow (I didn't enter the crazy competition there—talk about playing basketball with Michael Jordan). Dino helped me to get better. I was becoming invested in getting the part. I didn't understand how I could star in a TV show while doing a Vegas show every night, but I wanted to win this time. I started to believe I could act. I didn't care about a story. I was trying to play a brilliant, fat, divorced alcoholic, and all I had for experience was being fat.

Finally, after several callback auditions, the producer took me aside and said something like, "You're really good at all the hard stuff. The stuff none of the other people can do, you're great at. But you really aren't good at the easy stuff. The stuff we need done all the time, every show. You're just not good. We sure wish you could do the easy stuff."

The hard stuff on a diet is supposed to be dealing with the cravings and mustering the willpower to pass up all the foods you love. I had pizza in Brooklyn with Lou Reed, and I remember that night and that pizza—and now the same pizza is available in Vegas. But I don't need the pizza for the memory. The fabulous chef Jet Tila taught me to cook the best steak I've ever eaten, and I cooked a version on TV and the judges agreed it was the best steak ever, and now I know how to do it and how good it is, and I live in Vegas, the land of good steaks, but it's still not hard to resist.

I went to Krispy Kreme Doughnuts the day they opened in Las Vegas and got the first Vegas glazed raspberry-filled Krispy Kreme doughnuts and some cold milk and they were so good. I've had dozens and dozens, probably grosses of Krispy Kremes.

I had my mom's pork roast and homemade blueberry pie baked with shortening and blueberries she picked herself (she didn't pick the shortening herself). I had a Jet Tila steak. I ate Indian food with the prince of Sri Lanka. I had Chinese food at the best restaurant in Beijing (not as good as the pizza in New York with Lou Reed). I've had scallops on a dive boat, brought up from the bottom of the sea and served disgustingly fresh, almost live, with some wasabi right there on the boat. I've had my mom's macaroni and cheese with real Vermont cheddar. I've had one of Mrs. Teller's glorious meals with three different kinds of succulent meats and fresh bread and butter. I had the first Egg McMuffin served in Greenfield, Massachusetts, when I was in high school because I thought it was funny to stay up all night and be there when they opened.

No one is ever going to make a blueberry pie like my mom. I'm not ever going to have her gravy on Thanksgiving again. She and Lou Reed are dead and gone, and gravy without Mom is just salty liquid fat (sounds good), and pizza without the rock 'n' roll animal is just pizza. I can't live those memories again, so why not make new good memories?

I've had the lobster at Ruth's Chris Steak House, and wow, it's good. I've had several different cuts of their steaks served rare, bloody, and perfect. I've had their fully loaded baked potato and loved all of it. I had a "salad" that was dripping with blue cheese and bacon. I've had their chocolate mousse that I always seemed to have room for—another couple thousand fat calories.

What I'd never had was their plain steamed asparagus with a little fresh lemon squeezed on it and a plain, earthy baked potato without even oil to make it shiny. That was a different thing.

For almost sixty years I ate like a fucking hell-bent pig (my mom fed me pretty well). I've eaten sea urchin and fried chicken and waffles. I've had real maple sugar on snow in a sugarhouse in New England with my mom, my dad, and my sister. I've had some great eats. So for the next forty-five years, I'll make new memories. I'll have memories of eating things with my wife and children that will be new and tasty and allow me to maybe spend more healthy years with said wife and children.

I won't eat pizza with Lou Reed, but I have that memory. Maybe I'll get to eat a vegan meal with Paul McCartney—who knows?

As I write this, it seems like pure bullshit. The worst kind of resolution of cognitive dissonance. It's worse than sour grapes, it's boring steak; some grapes are really sour, but I never really had a steak that I didn't enjoy. So, I guess it is bullshit, but it's bullshit that feels right for me now.

I've had truffled macaroni and cheese with bacon at fancy-ass restaurants, and it didn't really bring me the comfort of my mom's macaroni and cheese. Why keep trying to chase that first high? That's heroin thinking. Nothing is going to be like the first Krispy Kreme I had with Teller in South Carolina, just two Yankee boys running away to be carny trash and getting our first taste of the sweet, fat South on our way to making magic. So, fuck it—let's have a potato.

LOSING IT! 74.5 POUNDS IN 83 DAYS (0.9 POUNDS A DAY, 24.4% OF BODY WEIGHT)

IT'S JUST A GODDAMN POTATO

We were going to eat nothing but potatoes. Nothing else. Nothing but potatoes. Just potatoes. Potatoes and nothing else.

Could we eat sweet potatoes?

Yes.

Could we eat baked potatoes?

Yes.

Could we eat fingerlings?

Yes.

Could we have a little nonfat sour cream?

No.

A little fake nonfat, unsalted butter?

No.

Broccoli was okay, right?

No.

Weird purple Japanese sweet potatoes?

Yes.

Boiled potatoes?

Yes.

Raw potatoes?

Yes.

Fried potatoes?

Of course—they're potatoes, right? NO, you asshole, oil has been added.

Peeled and mashed with nothing added?

No, you gotta eat the whole potato. Always. Skin and all, and all the water.

Can you slice them thin and microwave them to make them like chips?

No—I just said you gotta eat all the water.

Would this plan work with other food?

Yes, but you're not doing other foods, you're going to eat just potatoes.

Just potatoes?

Yes.

What the fuck?

Yes.

Okay, so, just potatoes. How many potatoes?

As many as you want.

How often?

As often as you want.

So, I can eat twenty potatoes in a day?

Yes.

Really?

Yes. Sure, eat thirty a day, but you won't.

He was so fucking smug. CrayRay acted like he knew every question before we asked it. He was condescending. I was a little fat ant, and he was king. He was our Potato King and knew everything that was going to happen, and we weren't fit to eat fingerlings off the bottoms of his boots.

I fell in love with him. I was no longer concerned about health or getting thin—I wanted to serve Master CrayRay. I'm not really much of the submissive type, but this was proof that we're all everything. We're all Master Grey and Don Johnson's daughter. (I didn't see the movie, but . . . I know what I'm talking about.)

Just potatoes. Yes, Master.

Why the goddamn potato? I didn't want to ask much about this at the time, but since then I've found out a bit more, so I'll tell you here. After all, you aren't in the cult . . . yet.

Part of it is my fault. A long time ago, Teller and I came up with our version of what is likely the oldest trick in magic, the Cups and Balls. We first did it four-handed with red plastic cups, and then we did it four-handed with clear plastic cups. This is what we claimed magicians got really mad at us for. In fact there were only a few middle-aged bullshit magicians who didn't understand what we were doing, but we played up their objections so we could act like victims. Some poor bastard would write in a mimeographed newsletter with a circulation of maybe a few hundred that Penn & Teller were giving away magic secrets and they shouldn't do that, and then we would pull the quotation out of context and give it to David Letterman to read as part of our introduction to a few million people, and we would come out acting like we were being persecuted by the magic establishment. Disingenuous, lying, manipulative, unfair assholes, that's us. And even with us doing the Cups and Balls with clear cups, you still couldn't follow it. It gave the trick away only if you already knew how the trick was done. My buddy Jerry Camaro did his own Cups and Balls during our intermission, after the whole audience had seen our Cups and Balls with clear cups, and still fooled the shit out of everyone.

Now, in the classic Cups and Balls, you want to have a final load that surprises the audience when you lift the last cup. Magicians had historically used baby chicks, but late-twentieth-century American audiences would be uncomfortable imagining how baby chicks would have to be handled in order to hide them on your body and sneak them quickly under a cup. When we had to come up with a final load, a big punch line for our version of the Cups and Balls, we knew ours had to be mundane. That was our style. We think cows are funny, so we also think potatoes are funny. And even in twenty-first-century America, no one seems to care how potatoes are treated. So instead of a baby chick, our final load was a potato. The line I said was, "And for our final load . . . it's a goddamn potato! It's just a goddamn potato!" That was the punch line to the whole bit.

CrayRay had seen our show a zillion times, and he always cracked up when I said, "It's just a goddamn potato!" When he immersed himself in nutrition and thought about doing a mono-diet to knock people out of their food-heads for two weeks, he had a lot of choices:

He could do corn. Two weeks of just corn.

Anything besides corn?

No.

Anything on the corn?

No.

As much as I want?

Yes.

Or he could have done beans. Two weeks of just beans.

Anything besides beans?

No.

Anything on the beans?

No.

As much as I want?

Yes.

But "It's just a goddamn potato!" kept ringing in CrayRay's head. It made him laugh every time he thought of feeding people "just a goddamn potato." It's so fucking stupid. And so pedestrian. And so easy to find and prepare. And so cheap. Now, beans would be funnier to some because of all the farting, but that's not really my kind of humor. To me, there's nothing funnier than a potato.

CrayRay also chose the potato as a fuck-you to other nutrition people. The potato is hated. CrayRay wanted to say fuck you to that diet, so potatoes were a good choice. He also wanted to say fuck you to the paleo people. And he said fuck you to them so well that if you search "Ray Cronise" and "Paleo," you will see a lot of Internet chatter about Ray and his potatoes. He drove the paleo people crazier than they already were. But if the paleo diet is really that good for you, how come the Flintstones need multivitamins?

So the goddamn potato was kinda sorta a little bit my fault. I could have been eating corn for two weeks. CrayRay chose it for the same kind of reason that P&T chose the three of clubs as our "force card." Early on Teller and I wanted to let the audience in on part of the magic. And we wanted to let people who saw us a lot in on more secrets than people who saw us only once or twice.

Artists are always looking for universals. Poets want to find the little things that we all share but don't yet know we share. My favorite living author is Nicholson Baker. I just love every single thing he writes. He breaks my heart, teaches me, scares me, makes me laugh, and gives me a joyful, bitter, sad, glorious reason to live. He's the best. In his first book, *The Mezzanine*, he covers every thought going through his narrator's head as he walks into his office building and onto the escalator. The whole book takes place during those few seconds. Every thought. There are footnotes, and it's just fabulous. And it's so real. Every thought seems like an exact thought this person would have. In the middle of the book, there's one thing he wrote that made me scream out loud. The narrator explains that every time he sees a bottle of vitamin C tablets, or even hears the phrase "vitamin C," he sings to himself a line from the Grateful Dead song "Truckin'" to himself. Every single time "vitamin C" comes into his consciousness, he sings, "Livin' on reds, vitamin C, and cocaine / All a friend can say is ain't it a shame." I don't like the Grateful Dead, not at all. I went to see Dylan and the Dead at the Meadowlands just to see what the fuss was about, and I ended up in Dylan's dressing room playing pinball with his son and waiting for Bob to go on while the Dead played through the walls. I like Phish okay, but I'm not a big jam-band guy. I have never done "reds" and don't really know what they are—speed, right? And I've never used cocaine, and I don't take vitamin C. So there's no reason that, like the narrator, that line should be in my head every time I hear the phrase "vitamin C," but it is, and Nicholson Baker (who is about the same age as me) nailed it. And that is pure poetry.

When Louis CK, Chris Rock, or George Carlin hit on something that we all think, it's just perfect. But magicians piss that away. They do everything they can to avoid universals. Everyone in a modern audience knows that magic is just tricks. Everyone in a modern audience knows the word "palm" means to hold something secretly in one's hand. And everyone knows that sometimes when a magician proffers a deck to have a single card freely selected, it's not always a free choice, and just about everyone knows the term for that is "force." Everyone knows that, and everyone knows that everyone knows that . . . except magicians. Magicians think common knowledge is deeply arcane. So, they pretend.

We wanted people to know that we knew that they knew, so we wanted to make sure that when we forced a card in nearly any of our performances (not all—sometimes we want to force a card and get away with it), we used the same card every time as a wink to those who like to think about our tricks a bit.

We needed a card that was clear and visible, so no court cards and no cards with a lot of pips—too hard to see from the back of the house. Black cards show up better than red cards, so that narrowed it down to ace through five, spades or clubs. Aces were out, because they rank highly in many card games. They're fancy-ass, and we're mundane, so fuck aces. Two is too close to the ace; it's the ace's loser suck-up. For some reason spades seemed just a little fancier to us than clubs. That got us to the three of clubs, which was perfect. The three of clubs seems like the humblest of cards. There's nothing special about it. Nothing at all. But it's visible, and it seems like a random card. And when that random card shows up every time P&T have a card freely selected . . . that strikes us as funny. We've had some success making this humble card a little better known. Lots of other magicians and even filmmakers have used the three of clubs as a little wink to us. Look for it. It shows up in the movie *Watchmen*, but it appears in a lot of other places, too. Ray wanted to do for the goddamn potato what we'd tried to do for the three of clubs.

So I was going to eat nothing but potatoes for two weeks.

EXERCISE—CLIMB MOUNT EVEREST FOR BUTTER

No meat, no fish, no bread, no butter, no pastry, no pasta, no cheese, no sugar, no milk, no oil, and no salt, but hey, no exercise!

Just add some oral sex to the right side of the equation and we've got parity. I can't promise you head (feel free to ask when you see me next), but even "no exercise" alone makes it pretty attractive. When CrayRay first offered me that upside (the "no exercise" upside—we haven't blown each other yet), I really couldn't believe it. Every other time I've tried to lose weight, exercise was always part of the package, and I really fucking hate exercise.

CrayRay kind of buried the lede. If he wanted to be a filthy-rich diet guru, he would have called his plan the No-Exercise Couch-Potato Diet. I don't even really need oral sex added to the mix to make that attractive to me. If CrayRay didn't throw in the no-exercise part in order to make a shit-ton of money, why did he do it? If I was losing almost a pound a day for three months without exercising, wouldn't I have lost even more if I'd thrown in a jog or two?

CrayRay says no, that weight loss and muscle building (that's what exercise does, build muscles) are two very different things. CrayRay's books and papers explain the no-exercise part of the plan in language like this: "Losing excess adipose tissue and gaining muscle are two completely different physiologies. Weight loss requires a restriction, or deficit. Muscle gain requires fuel and nutrients to support activity and the repair of tissue. Hypertrophy happens when one stresses the muscle, tearing down tissue. Through a process called hormesis, the tissue grows back stronger after the stress."

Exercise is for bodybuilding, and I had more than enough body— about a third more body than was good for me. What I needed was a building moratorium. I wouldn't get out of exercise forever. Exercise is important for good health. But I wouldn't do any until I hit target weight. Exercise wouldn't help me with weight loss; I couldn't outrun my mouth.

There are people who exercise enough that they need to stuff in as many calories as they can. Before his little Olympic swim meets, Michael Phelps would have a breakfast that included three sandwiches of fried eggs, cheese, lettuce, tomato, fried onions, and mayonnaise; an omelet; a bowl of grits; three slices of French toast with powdered sugar; and three chocolate-chip pancakes. I would do fifteen push-ups and run on a treadmill for twenty minutes and figure that if Mike could eat that, I could at least have some oatmeal. And a glass of orange juice. A big glass. And maybe a couple of eggs, and some toast with . . . ice cream. Jesus, I had a good workout, so I'll need a good lunch; gotta get that protein in me so I don't lose muscle mass.

Friends of mine leave their little workouts and go to meetings with a Tupperware container filled with skinless "low-fat" chicken breasts and fruit. They think they're eating healthy. They just did an hour with their buff trainer, and now they're building body mass—muscle and fat, and they already have plenty of fat. That's the problem.

I understand immediately why people collect stamps. I understand why people play polo. I can relate to every sexual kink I've ever
seen video of. It makes sense that people would build copies of the
Great Wall of China with matchsticks (do they?), set up a million
dominoes, or learn to solve a Rubik's Cube blindfolded underwater,
execute a perfect shuffle, or how to click-speak !Kung. But it took
me a long time to have an inkling why anyone would climb Everest.
"Because it's there" is bullshit. It's cold, you can't breathe, you can
die, and there's spotty Wi-Fi. Then I either read or made up that the
people on Everest have trouble getting enough calories. While the
frost is biting off their toes, they have to eat sticks of butter to try
to get enough energy for their bodies. Hey now! Now we're talking.
Maybe people climb Everest just to eat sticks of butter. When I was
craving fat and salt all the time, eating butter sounded pretty good.
Call Tenzing Norgay.

In my warm, cozy local gym, I would plug my weight and age
into the elliptical machine to see how many calories' worth of butter
I could eat after the workout. The number of calories the machine
shows is a very high estimate of total calories burned during the workout, not the difference between calories burned exercising and calories
burned sitting like a lump. I could burn most of those estimated calories reading the *Times* on my iPad. Saying that is already making the
skeptic's mistake of trying to figure out how we twist the numbers to
make them bullshit. The fact is, most bullshit is just bullshit to start
with. I have no real evidence that the calorie number on the elliptical
machine has anything to do with what my body is really burning. All
that number ever did for me was give me license to have a scone at
Bucky's. Yeah, the exercise gave me tone, but it also made me hungry.
It made me more likely to fail at whatever jive-ass diet I was trying to
follow at the time. I've finally realized it's better to just not eat butter
and stay away from Chomolungma.

If you really care about the science of this stuff, you'll read CrayRay's book. There are all sorts of things the body does during mild exercise to hang on to fat, and I (and my sweaty friends wearing their stupid shorts in their home gyms) never did more than *mild* exercise. Yeah, I used to swim for half an hour a day, but that didn't make me Michael Phelps swimming uphill on Everest.

All over the country there are atheist billboards. The billboards feature stuff like Thomas Jefferson quotations and pro-LGBT (Michael Phelps's breakfast sandwich—Lettuce, Guacamole, Bacon, and Tomato) greetings from the atheist community. Some of them are really sweet, like just wishing a Merry Christmas and Happy Chanukah from all of us heathens. I'm hoping we can get more surreal with these messages. I would love to see a billboard that just says JESUS HAD A SWIMMER'S BODY. I can't really defend this with comedic theory, but it sure makes me laugh my newly skinny ass off. It brings the theological debate to where it belongs.

I used to swim every day. There's a big lap pool at the Slammer. For half an hour every day I swam hard, but I never had a swimmer's body like our Lord Jesus Christ. I didn't get thin until I stopped exercising. But I didn't stop exercising for life. The week after I hit my target weight, I went back to exercise. Not Norgay/Phelps–type exercise, just enough to build my body back up a bit. When people talk to me about my weight loss, they always seem to end up asking in horror, "Didn't you lose some muscle mass?" I was supposed to keep one hundred extra pounds of fat on my body just so I wouldn't lose an inch around my biceps? Yeah, I lost weight everywhere (except my cock, motherfucker!). Even my stupid head got smaller. I had to adjust my hats. My arms and legs got pretty thin by the time I hit my target weight. The first time I exercised after hitting my target, I struggled to do three push-ups with bad form. As a fat fuck I could bang out fifteen and then huff and puff for several minutes.

The exercise I chose to do after I hit my target was the seven-minute workout I first read about in the *Times*. I picked one of the zillions of apps to talk me through it on my phone. The *NYT* ran a few articles about how you can exercise your ass off for just seven minutes and be done with it. Twelve exercises for thirty seconds each, with ten seconds' "rest" (they call it rest—assholes!) between each one. I used to say I didn't mind exercise—it was just that it took so much time out of my busy day (most of that busy day spent fantasizing about eating butter on Sagarmāthā and looking up more local names for Everest). The *NYT* called my bluff: it wasn't just the time; I hated exercise when I was fat. Now that I'm at my target weight, now that I'm thinner, it's not that bad. My seven minutes go by pretty fast. I went from barely being able to do three push-ups to banging out fifteen in thirty seconds with no problem. It took just a few weeks of doing seven minutes every other day. That was about twenty-five minutes a week! After a month I added ten minutes of free weights after my seven minutes to fill up a little of the loose skin on my biceps and triceps. That worked really fast. At my target weight, my muscles grew really fast with exercise. Working out seems to work when I'm not eating butter. I don't really know what that means, but it also seemed like it was better muscle I was building. When I exercised when I was fat, it felt like I was building marbled-prime-rib-type muscle, muscle full of fat. After losing all that weight with no exercise, I sure lost a lot of size on my arms. But when I exercise now, it feels like I'm building lean muscle. The muscle on my arms looks really different. There's a shape to my muscle that makes it look like muscle. I've never had that before. I had big arms—fairly strong arms—but it seemed like they were made of sloppy fat muscle. Now they seem like they're made of clean muscle. Remember, I have no idea what really happened to me. But that's how it feels.

The whole world seems to scream that the way to lose weight

and be healthy is to eat frequent protein-rich meals and to exercise. CrayRay says that's the way to gain weight (muscle). That's body-building, and when I look around at all the people I know who are doing that, it sure seems like they're all fat. CrayRay's plan goes against all the popular, contemporary conventional wisdom. I honestly meant it when I wrote that I don't know jack shit in the disclaimer at the beginning of this book. I am one data point. I don't even know if any of what I did "worked" for me. It could be that while I was doing everything CrayRay told me to do, I lost weight for some other magical reason. It could be that if I'd exercised while I was doing all this, I would have lost more weight and been even healthier. It sure doesn't seem that way. It sure seems like CrayRay is right, but I don't know. I know about a dozen people have followed me into this cult and it *seemed* to work the same for them, but we're still a very small sample. If CrayRay makes some money from his book or gets some funding, he'll continue his real science. CrayRay is learning about this shit. He's doing experiments with controls and getting real data. He's learning shit.

I know I lost one hundred pounds, and I'm reporting what was going on with me while that weight went away. But it's possible that I might have been better off climbing Everest and eating a stick of butter every two hours. There's a lot of protein in butter.

POTATOES ARE REALLY GOOD

I had hoped that Goudeau and I would start gobbling potatoes right away, but CrayRay wouldn't let us. He needed the timing to be perfect. He told us that days three and four of the potato famine can be really tough, that we might feel like shit. He said we couldn't really work during that time, or have any important engagements. He said most people start on a Thursday so that those bad potato days fall on the weekend and don't fuck up their work.

Well, I work all the time, so there was no way to schedule the potato famine around time off. But I could schedule it around the nights Penn & Teller don't have shows in Vegas. Thursday and Friday are our dark days. "Wait just a fucking minute—you're in showbiz and you take Friday off?" But Friday isn't magic in Vegas. Saturday is. We sell out Saturdays. But Friday is when most people arrive in Vegas, and the thinking is that they'll have supper and throw a fuck into their date or something, but probably won't see a show. Fridays are special in other cities, where people are home and don't have to travel, so they go out to shows on Fridays. And since we're dark in Vegas on Fridays, we can do one-nighters in other cities on our dark days. So even our days off are chosen with greed in mind.

Thursday and Friday, December 11 and 12, 2014, were rarities for P&T: we didn't have shows in Vegas, and we didn't have shows on the road. On top of that, my whole family was away visiting Grandpa that week. I had writing to do (I always have writing to do) and some meetings, but no really difficult work and no social obligations. I could stay home and starve and hate potatoes. Goudeau would do the time with me.

We decided that Goudeau and Penn would eat nothing but potatoes for two weeks starting at 12:01 a.m. on Tuesday, December 9. CrayRay gave us a lot of other rules. We were supposed to sleep a lot. We had to allow ourselves to be cold. And we were not to exercise. Yup—we were going to lose weight by sleeping, not exercising, and eating all the potatoes we wanted. No doubt, we had joined a crazy cult.

According to CrayRay, humans, or at least Americans, have eliminated winter. We have conquered the three realms that control all other undomesticated animals' lives: light, heat, and food. We are bright, warm, and fed all year round. There aren't really seasons for us anymore. But CrayRay believes seasons matter. We spend bright, warm, fed time preparing for a winter that never comes. CrayRay wanted Penn and Goudeau to experience ninety days of winter so we could use some of the fat we'd saved up. He wanted us cold, hungry, healthy, and happy.

I didn't understand much of this at the time, and I still don't understand a lot of it, but CrayRay's two-week potato famine was designed to knock our asses out of the American relationship with food. CrayRay said most diets fail because people can do anything for ninety days, but then they crack. People can change how they eat for a season, but that's about it. So, if you diet like a grown-up and lose two pounds a week by eating sensibly, you lose about twenty-five pounds. You can see and feel twenty-five pounds, but it doesn't blow your mind. Losing twenty-five pounds is not life-changing if you need to lose over thirty, and if you don't need to lose over thirty, you probably don't need such a radical diet. So, you can slowly and sensibly lose twenty-five pounds over twelve weeks, and then say "Fuck it" and slowly put it back on.

CrayRay's idea was to have us lose weight so fast that we would feel it every day. He promised us six-tenths to eight-tenths of a pound a day, which is four to five and a half pounds a week! After twelve weeks we'd be down sixty pounds, and we would really be able to see and feel that. At that point our diet would change to whole plants, including nuts and fruit. The new diet would feel like a feast. He would restrict us so much that after we'd gotten used to eating no animal products, salt, oil, or refined grains, it would seem like Thanksgiving to have an orange.

Two weeks of nothing but potatoes also eliminates eating both as a social activity and as entertainment. Eating just potatoes means you eat only when you feel like you really need to eat. There's no entertainment in a potato. And it's not social. You don't sit around with friends at a plain potato bar.

It also eliminates what CrayRay loosely calls "addiction." Two weeks of potatoes would enable us to taste smaller amounts of salt and fat than we ever could with our Standard American Diet (called, for all sorts of reasons, SAD). We would see our culture from the outside a little bit. We would see billboards dripping cheese and people eating big muffins in business meetings. We would see everyone else eating constantly. We would be knocked out of our heads. Two weeks of nothing but potatoes would reboot my eating. I was going to leave all my old food habits behind. All the stuff I knew about myself and food would change. I was so ready for this.

The rules were simple: For two full weeks I would eat nothing but potatoes. Just potatoes, nothing added. And nothing taken away—skin and all. Sweet potatoes are potatoes! Wow. Fingerling, Idaho, russet, red, new, any kind of potato I wanted. I could microwave them or bake them or boil them or eat them raw. As many as I wanted, any time I wanted—but just potatoes. I could put some pepper on them, but no salt, no Tabasco, nothing. I would eat potatoes for two weeks. No ketchup. No vinegar. Just potatoes. I would be an old-fashioned meat and potatoes guy without the meat.

DAY 1: 304.3 POUNDS

I weighed myself on my fancy Withings scale: 304.3 pounds. CrayRay insists on the Withings; every morning, right before my shower, I step on the scale. It weighs me, takes my pulse, measures my fat content, monitors the air quality, and tells me if it's going to rain. You think that's a joke, right? You think I added "tells me if it's going to rain" as a joke, like it's a floor wax and a dessert topping, but I'm not kidding—it measures all that. *And* it stores the information on the Internet and graphs it and sends it to my phone and to CrayRay's phone. Our leader would know every time I stepped on the scale. Thank you, Withings. And that last sentence wasn't a joke, either.

I got home from the show that Monday night to find that EZ had boiled potatoes for me. Up until this point, I'd been trying to eat kind of healthy, so after the show at the theater I'd have a big piece of broiled salmon, some broccoli, and some spinach. I thought broiled salmon was kind of safe-healthy, but CrayRay said, "It's just fat. Think of it as just a slab of fat. You don't need another animal's fat. You can use your own." So that Monday night I canceled my room-service order and drove home and had a potato. I couldn't remember the last time I'd eaten a plain potato. Maybe never? I took a bite. Without the butter and salt, I could kind of taste the potato. It had a nice, dirty taste and smell, and I found comfort in it. I would soon come to know everything about the taste of potatoes, but this was the first one.

With a nice potato on board, I watched *Black Mirror* with my wife, and then had a sweet potato before taking my bath. To give you an idea of what a change this was, most nights, after having my salmon and watching a little TV, my before-bath snack was some really sharp cheddar cheese dipped in peanut butter, accompanied by a couple of Saltines. See? This was a big diet change.

I read in the bathtub. I told you I would write about my experience of weight loss. I was reading Norman Mailer's *The Executioner's Song* and loving it. An amazing book, and even better when read in a hot tub of water very early on a beautiful desert morning.

I woke up feeling great. I often felt sluggish in the morning, but maybe having less salt and fat on board helped. I don't know. Or maybe it was all psychosomatic. But I stepped on the scale, and . . .

. . . I'd lost 1.8 pounds. And I'd eaten normally for most of that day. Call it "water weight," call it whatever you want, but I was 1.8 pounds lighter. Getting that immediate reinforcement really meant something. I got up and did not exercise. I microwaved a couple of potatoes, both sweet and regular, wrapped them in tin foil, threw them in my car, and headed over to meet Goudeau for coffee. We were allowed all the coffee we wanted—black with no sugar, but all we wanted. I've been off caffeine for decades, so I was just drinking dirty water.

I went to the P&T rehearsal at the theater and worked with Piff the Magic Dragon, Johnny Thompson, our great crew, and Teller. I felt great and really energetic, and we got a lot done.

I came home and had supper with my family. Roast chicken for them, potatoes for me. But the children joined in with me. They like to eat what Daddy eats. I had a couple of potatoes but wasn't sated, so when I got to the theater I had another potato, and then the show started.

Now, one of the most important parts of this CrayRay diet is no exercise. But I was still doing the full P&T show. It's not a lot of exercise, but it's more than you think. I move a lot onstage and talk really loudly for a long time. I also concentrate. Even after doing P&T shows for forty years, I can't coast. I really can't. I can do part of the show on autopilot, and my autopilot works great—some of the best moments in our shows have happened while I was thinking about other stuff—but I can't do the whole show on autopilot. It takes a lot of thinking. We do things in our show that are dependent on audience members. We perform some proudly fake mind reading, but even though it's fake, it's different every night.

About halfway through the show, I began to feel like shit. I started flop-sweating and felt like I was going to throw up. I was light-headed and distracted, right on the edge of fainting. This wasn't good. I had friends in the audience. Later they said the show looked great. I don't think Teller knew, but I was missing my 1.8 pounds, and I was missing eating food that wasn't potatoes. I was just coming up on twenty-four hours of the potato famine. This might be a long two weeks. I hadn't really told CrayRay how sick I was at the start; even though I had been in the hospital, I don't think *I* even realized how sick I was. We still don't understand everything that was going on, but the very drugs that had kept me alive as a sick person were poisoning the healthier person I was becoming. I was losing weight so quickly that I was a different patient from week to week. My doctor was rushing to keep up with my health and to take me off the meds at the right time. This was why I needed my doctor on board every step of the way.

Our show was followed by MovieNight. MovieNight started in NYC when we were playing Off-Broadway. A bunch of us would meet after the show at Howard Johnson's in Times Square, have a snack, and then go to a movie. There were two rules for choosing what to see: the start time had to be close to midnight, and the movie had to be the most likely to go away quickly. When *Rolling Stone* wrote about MovieNight, they thought we were just trying to see bad movies. No—there are just a lot of bad movies. We'd give a round of polite golf applause whenever the name of the film was spoken in the movie, and we'd sometimes say "Wow" when the title of another movie was spoken in a movie, as in "Help, Dad, do the right thing." Wow, wow, wow.

When MovieNight moved to Vegas, it got weirder. It moved from public theaters to my house, and changed from MovieNight to Bacon MovieNight. To choose the movie, we used the theory behind Six Degrees of Kevin Bacon: that night's movie had to be connected to the last one we'd watched through an actor. Bacon became as important as the movie, maybe more so. One MovieNight during the potato famine, a few people decided to create a MovieNighter ritual. The MovieNight nurse decided she should have her naked ass spanked with bacon. Who am I to blow against the wind? Some MovieNighters shot video of the heathen baptism, and took turns whacking her with the bacon. Then they fried it up. I could have eaten baptism ass bacon. There were also bacon-wrapped dates with Gorgonzola, a big pepperoni pizza, guacamole, home-made brownies, and popcorn, both cheese-flavored and buttered. I love all those foods. I ate a potato. When my friends asked, "What's with the potato?" I answered just like I should: "This potato means fuck you." That's a perfectly acceptable MovieNight answer, and all my friends understood.

Ray's instruction was to not talk to anyone about this. Everyone has theories on diet, and they will try to help. I'm fully aware that big parts of this plan might be bullshit, but I joined the cult. It's pretty funny. If you decide to take a quick ride on a motorcycle or eat nothing but candy for a week, your friends aren't going to say anything—but try eating a little different, and everyone will be on your dick. Is eating only potatoes crazy? Yes. Is it life-threatening? No. Should anyone care? Especially the fat fucks all around you stuffing their faces with candy and French fries? Fuck them. Shut up. I'll cut to the chase: the potato means fuck you, and we're done.

DAY 2: 302.5

The show was really hard. I mean *really* hard. I was flop-sweating and felt light-headed and faint. The audience didn't know, but man, I knew. I don't want to gloss over this. I love all the changes I made to my health and my diet, but an important part of CrayRay's program is no exercise, and I was still doing the show through the whole thing. I'm not doing a Cirque du SoWhat act; I'm not an acrobat, and I'm not crowd-surfing or running around at random like Springsteen. I'm mostly just talking. But I'm talking loudly, and that seems to take some energy; I'm also keeping a lot in my head, at least for me. The P&T script is around a hundred pages of dialogue, and it's all me. Also there's a lot of the show that changes every night—audience members' names and so on—and parts of the show are flow-charted, so there are different lines and actions depending on what happens. It takes a lot of focus.

The other thing that seems to make a difference is that comedy is . . . timing. So, I have to judge my timing based on the audience, the magic, and Teller. I can't do it based on how I feel. So if I were to get just a tiny bit light-headed out in the world, I would just take a breath, or even sit down for five seconds. At any other time in my life, I could do that—but not during the show. There's no place during any line of the show where I can take an extra breath without hurting the performance. And it's only during Teller's stupid Red Ball and Silverfish tricks that I can even sit down for a few seconds.

Let me be clear on this: I am not saying that I work hard. I don't. Not at all. I'm in showbiz. But I do get light-headed when I'm eating only potatoes. This feeling kept up for the whole ninety days, and even occasionally after. CrayRay and I tried all sorts of things to keep me from getting light-headed. We added a metric shit-ton of rice once I was finished eating only potatoes. I even bought some of those diabetic glucose pills and ate them while Teller was out doing his fancy Red Ball trick. I would sit down and eat sugar and hope that I wouldn't get light-headed. But I still did. We never really solved this problem, but the upside was worth a little light-headedness.

DAY 3: 296.2

Look at those numbers. On the second day alone I lost almost five pounds. And by day three I'd lost over eight pounds total. If you stop eating salt, you do lose a lot of water weight. It wasn't all fat. Maybe not even mostly fat. But it was still weight I wasn't carrying around with me.

CrayRay had warned me that days three and four are the hardest, and my potato schedule was built around those. They were Thursday and Friday, and I had those days off. It wasn't terrible. I was just quiet and sleepy. They were gentle days. Not days of suffering but days of sitting quietly and taking naps. It was kind of like being sick without the being sick part. I liked it. I liked days three and four; they were a gentle, quiet time-out.

DAY 6: 290.0

At this point I was averaging more than two pounds a day.

By now I've watched a lot of friends go through the potato famine.

It's pretty remarkable. With the exception of Theresa Goudeau, every-one has found it easier than expected. But my buddy Theresa had a really hard time. She got sick and couldn't keep the potatoes down. That's why I keep making it clear that I'm writing *only* about my expe-rience. I didn't run a scientific experiment. I didn't set up controls and other stuff I don't really understand. I'm just a dipshit potato-eater who lost a lot of weight.

One of the things the potato famine did was pull me out of the food culture. I've never drunk alcohol or done drugs, so when I walk into a bar or a rave (which I don't do often), I see it through sober eyes. I have a buddy who was high all the time. He made a documen-tary about drugs for TV and had to produce and direct, so he had to work sober in a lot of places where he had once been high and party-ing. It blew his mind. He didn't think he could drink and do drugs ever again (I think he managed to get over that). But when you're losing weight and eating potatoes and nothing else, the food culture seems so batshit crazy.

I would go into Hollywood meetings at eleven o'clock in the morning and there would be food in the conference room. Who at that meeting was honestly going to be hungry? And of those people who were hungry, who couldn't wait through the meeting for lunch at noon? Muffins are everywhere. The ads for food that wallpaper our world and flood our senses are invisible until you're just eating pota-toes. CrayRay points out that our lives are one big meal interrupted by a little work, occasional fucking, and watching TV.

CrayRay has the real info, but I was losing weight on potatoes at the same rate I would have lost weight on a water fast. Eating potatoes was pretty much the same as not eating at all. But I think eating po-tatoes blew my mind more than not eating at all. It took all the enter-tainment out of eating. It took all the habit out of eating. No one just hands you a potato like they would a doughnut or a muffin. They aren't available in every single store. You have to think about getting potatoes.

I also learned that "hot potato" is a very good image. A baked potato fresh out of the microwave or oven is so fucking hot. I'm a fire-eater and am used to burning my mouth, but potatoes are so much more dangerous than torches. Potatoes taught me about our culture of food, and they taught me about patience. Eating only potatoes taught me to wait before sticking that soft soldering iron in my mouth. I also learned that having a hot potato in your pocket is really fun. The perfect hand warmer. As I write this, I want to go back to potato time. Life is simple when you're just eating potatoes.

During my potato time I would get automated e-mails from CrayRay—mostly cheerleader-y stuff, some science stuff, and a lot of cult stuff. A lot of stuff designed to suck me into his world. It was around day six that CrayRay had me start my "contrast showers." You've been thinking that eating only potatoes isn't a very exciting cult, right? Well, this is when it got exciting.

CrayRay is not the potato guru. CrayRay is the *cold* guru. Most of CrayRay's experiments deal with cold. He is obsessed with the idea that we've conquered winter, and that it's a bad thing. We've conquered cold, dark, and hunger. We are always in summer. Everything is warm, bright, and bountiful. We live in paradise, but our bodies don't know that. Our bodies don't know summer is going to go on forever, so they keep saving up for a winter that never comes. CrayRay wants winter to come.

So for me, the summer of Big Macs and doughnuts had given way to potato winter. It's pretty close to what our ancestors would have had to eat in the winter: stored starches. CrayRay wanted me to be cold. Really cold. Not insane cold, like sitting in snow and taking ice baths, but really cold for me. So I got a timer app for my phone and put it in a plastic bag so I could take it into the shower.

Using the timer app, I'd allow myself ten seconds of warm shower, and when it beeped, I'd spin the control to as cold as it would go for twenty seconds. When it beeped again, I'd go back to warm for ten seconds. I did that ten times. So I spent five minutes going from hot to cold, back and forth, always longer in the cold than in the hot. I was in winter. It shocks the body. After the last hot, I'd go to cold for as long as I could stand. There are some magic tricks that are accomplished by memorizing things in order, and you need to be able to manipulate these . . . oh, let's say fifty-two things in your head to make the trick work. It takes a lot of practice. So I would run the most difficult mental exercise with these fifty-two "things" of four suits during that last blast of cold and have to get it all correct before I could turn the cold water off. Motherfucker!

CrayRay said the contrast showers would help me burn fat and change my mood. He said I would be invigorated. He said I would be happier. He said I would feel great.

The asshole was right. This was just crazy. I was hungry, cold, healthy, and happy. Wow.

DAY 7: 291.1

I went up. CrayRay said no big deal. I say fuck him.

DAY 11: 286.6

I'm jumping from day seven to day eleven because I want this all to be fair and accurate. I had to go to L.A. to do some business, and the fancy hotel I stayed at had a scale in the room, but I don't trust anything but my Withings scale. I wanted my tattletale Withings that runs to CrayRay and tells him everything about me every time I step on it. That's what I want. So although I jumped on the scale in L.A.

and things looked like they were kinda sorta on track, it's not good for this book. I want Withings or nothing! So that data isn't in here.

It was my first trip away from home and potatoes. It was really wonderful to go to the airport and not eat. I fly a lot, and airports and planes were always about eating shitty food and feeling terrible. I'd walk past Cinnabon to get a big fat muffin at Bucky's. I didn't have a Whopper with cheese and extra mayonnaise, but I'd grab some salty, spicy peanuts from the nut store. It's a nut and a legume—it's a pea nut. And on top of that, I'd eat shitty plane food. Of course, the Southwest Airlines jump to L.A. doesn't serve anything but peanuts and pretzels, but I sure used to eat them all.

I found that flying on this diet is the best. Eating on a plane is supposed to be a distraction. It's an activity. It doesn't matter that the food is shitty, it's something to do. Except it does matter. And there are better distractions that aren't really distractions but life. There are things I can do on a plane that I really want to do. Maybe you had to eat shit while sitting in a cramped area as a distraction before you had a smartphone, but now? There's no reason. I read the news, or a novel, or listen to Bob Dylan over and over. If it's a long trip and I have some room, I can work on my writing. Without food, flying is just an excuse to read and write and have time to myself. This diet I was on was amazing. All the stuff that I thought would be the hardest was the easiest. All the bugs were actually features. Not eating at airports and on planes is the greatest. I love it.

A word about pepper: It was allowed, but not until the second week, and even then I couldn't go nuts. CrayRay didn't want it at all that first week. Just taste the potato! And no Tabasco—that has too much flavor and just a little salt, and that's too much. Now when I go back to my potato buddies, I always have Tabasco, but in the early days of the potato famine, there was no reason for it. Just train yourself to notice the real tastes; don't blow your taste buds out. So I had a little black pepper, a bag of potatoes of all kinds, and a rock 'n' roll microwave. It might be the same microwave that Steven Tyler uses for his potatoes when he stays at that hotel.

That night I had a date with my wife to see Tim Minchin. Tim wrote the music and lyrics to the Roald Dahl show *Matilda the Musical*. He won every award in the world for that, and made all the money in the world. I think he's even better on his own as a performer, comedian, singer, and piano player. He's a hard-core skeptic and atheist, and his show isn't shy about that. Teller and I saw him with a full orchestra at the O_2 Arena in London, and he's wonderful. He's a good guy, too. I love Tim Minchin, and my wife seems to love me. She seems to love me a lot, but not compared to how much she loves Tim Minchin. The love my wife has for Tim is something that has to be experienced to be believed. From his Alice Cooper eyes to his Black Crowes bare feet, she loves every inch of this man. I love him, too, but there is no greater love than the love my wife has for Tim. It's the love Coltrane was carrying on about. Really something.

Tim was appearing at a show for the charity that Ryan Bell, the preacher who gave up god for a year, founded. I don't mean to ruin the surprise for you, but after that year, Ryan never went back. He works for a charity that helps the homeless, and this was a mostly atheist charity event where Tim was playing and Ryan was present. Also there was another one of my favorite comedy acts, Garfunkel and Oates. These two women are so funny and so charming. They weren't performing—they were in the audience, and my heart was pounding when I met them. I love them. Let EZ have Tim, and I'll take Garfunkel and Oates. If you can broker that deal, let me know.

So, the little after-show party was filled with people I knew and wanted to know. I was hobnobbing with my fellow wizards. They had white wine, and I had a Tupperware container full of fingerlings that EZ's mother had brought me. I was offering potatoes like hors d'oeuvres, and people were taking them.

"Hey, Tim, that was a great set, man, you are the best—want a potato?"

"A potato? Sure."

"Oh, man, I love Garfunkel and Oates, you guys just kill me. And I love the height difference; I like my two-person groups to have a height difference. Want a potato?"

"A potato? Sure."

The whole gang of charity atheist celebrities was eating potatoes. This could be the new thing. I didn't tell anyone about the diet. I was just a guy who carried potatoes around.

The next day in L.A., we shot a Mazda commercial. Commercial people know how to treat "talent," as we are fancifully called. My trailer was filled with all sorts of great snacks, and there was a food truck and a snack table that's called "craft services." Great snacks everywhere. I had a bag of potatoes.

I had been on the potato famine for about ten days, and already there was trouble. My suit didn't fit right. The wardrobe people had to do some pinning and adjusting. But commercial shoots are all about tiny adjustments. They had the Mazda there, and it's a beautiful car to begin with, but man, they made it just perfect. It was waxed and buffed and perfectly lit. They had been working on this commercial for days before our arrival. It had been months in the planning, but they were in this studio, lighting and working with P&T stand-ins, for days. They had shot the commercial a zillion times already. All that was left was to bring us in to fuck it up. We were sawing the car in half—that was the gag—and I would pretend to push the car apart (it was actually done mechanically), and the instant they said "Cut!" some guy would run in and buff the car everywhere I'd touched it and clean the floor everywhere that I'd moved my feet. It's amazing to see people who are that good at their jobs.

I had nothing to do. I just stood where they told me to stand and looked where they told me to look. Teller had to pull a lot of cloth out of his pocket, and we had to wave it around, which took several takes to get perfect, but every time I heard "Cut!" people would run in to buff, clean, and offer us sips of water, in case we had gotten parched standing there saying nothing in an air-conditioned room for fifteen seconds. They learned fast, soon adding, "Penn, would you like a potato?" to the litany. It turned out that I could go fifteen seconds without eating.

I learned something interesting during the shoot. Our TV and movie manager is my buddy Pete Golden. He's a surfer dude. The rumor about him is that he went to high school with Sean Penn, and the character of Jeff Spicoli is based on him. Maybe it's true, maybe it's not. He's a little younger than me, but not much, and he looks great—way better than me. Pete is slim and healthy. He saw me eating potatoes and said, "Oh, man, I love potatoes. When I'm on the road, I order a plain baked potato from room service and just have that for my dinner. I love them spuds, man." The joke we'd always had was that Pete didn't eat. We'd go to business lunches, and he would just order a salad and push it around on the plate. Or maybe he'd get a cheeseburger and then take one bite. It turns out that he would then go back to his room and have a potato. He also still surfs, so he gets all that CrayRay cold stuff every day in the water. He never talked about diet, but he's a potato brother. Amazing. There's a secret order of the potato. I wonder if I'm breaking some huge bond by writing about it in a book.

Besides shooting the commercial, I was doing other L.A. things, and one of the things I do in L.A. is pitch. My buddy Jesse Dylan once said that every Hollywood meeting took two months out of his life. I'm not sure exactly what that means, but I know it's true. We did a show in England called *Penn & Teller: Fool Us*, and it sure seemed like it did really well, but it was a big fancy expensive Saturday-night show and didn't do well enough, I guess, so we just did one season in the UK, and then the USA bought it; and then the UK bought the USA version after the USA bought the UK version and it did well. Showbiz. Pete, the potato eater, worked on selling it in the USA, and after a few years, the CW finally took a chance on us, and the show did really well for them. All of a sudden we had a TV show in the US again. Our last big successful show was *Bullshit!* and this one was *FU*. There's a theme in our titles. Since the CW liked me, I decided to try to sell them another crazy idea. This was a very hard sell. I'm a magician, a juggler, and, I guess, a comedian and author—but I'm not a TV writer, and I had an idea for a scripted one-hour . . . well, drama. Could *FU* have made them love me enough to consider letting me create and write a real show?

Pete had done his part of the job, and we had a lunch meeting with the big cheeses from the CW. The big secret in showbiz is that the "suits" are okay. I tend to like them. It's middle management in any corporation that has all the stress and ends up sometimes seeming like assholes, but the big bosses are usually okay.

I was into my second week of the potato famine, and they wanted to meet at Morton's. I was having a lunch meeting at a great steak house, and I was going to eat . . . a potato? I thought about that, and it didn't seem right. The potato is supposed to pull me out of social eating. But the potato would call attention to itself. It was potatoes or nothing, so I decided on nothing. Showbiz is my job. I was working. And, you know, I don't eat while I work. That's one of the things I wanted to break. I wasn't going to Morton's because I was hungry, I was going to Morton's to try to get some people to do a TV show with me. Why would I eat? I needed to be able to talk a lot and to focus, so why would I eat? We sat down, and everyone ordered. I ordered a big bottle of carbonated water and a big pot of decaffeinated coffee. I told them I wasn't hungry. No one freaked out. Who cares? It was at that moment I realized that part of the reason I was a fat fuck was because I'm a greedy fuck. I haven't admitted this to anyone, but sitting here all alone at my keyboard, it's a bit easier to be honest. One of the reasons I was a fat fuck was because other people were paying. I didn't grow up poor, but I didn't grow up rich. I grew up in a family where going out to eat was kind of a big deal, and going out for a steak or lobster was a very, very big deal. When I first got into showbiz, it was such a treat when someone would take us out for a meeting and pay for supper. It was amazing to be at a nice place and not be paying.

You would think that I now have a good-enough income that free food wouldn't matter much, but I'm still carny trash. I hadn't gotten rich enough to take away the lure, but I finally had gotten fat enough. I was finally too fat to take free meals. As embarrassing as it is to admit, it's true that it was a little hard for me to go out to lunch on a network expense account and have only fizzy water and coffee. Yeah, that's the kind of asshole I am. Here's the punch line: it was the best pitch I've ever done. I was totally working. I was focused on my idea, watching what they understood and seeing what I needed to explain better. I was able to pay attention to their expressions and let them provide input on my idea. I wasn't worried about cutting my steak or talking while I was chewing and spitting on the suit during a passionate moment. It was my best pitch—but is the show on the air? Well, you see, I've never gotten a drama on the air, so . . . it could be my best pitch, but still not good enough. But, as I write this, they haven't said no yet.

Days 10 and 11 were a different kind of potato famine test. This wasn't work, this was purely social. I was hanging with my troops in L.A. These are my real buddies. There were four of us: Richie Rich

Nathanson, an L.A. writer I know from MovieNight in NYC, who's since written for *Bullshit!* and become one of my dearest friends; Dino Cameron, now an LA director and writer, but you still know him as Chainsaw in *Summer School*; me; and finishing up the group was my new friend of only a couple of decades, Andy Lerner, another L.A. writer who used to be a radio commercial producer. He'd booked me to do a great Nestea Cool Iced Tea ad in which I'm bobbing for French fries in hot oil and being cooled off by Cool Iced Tea. The ad was pulled because someone thought people would be stupid enough to try it. We were all sitting at a Bucky's in Burbank, making jokes and complaining, and it got to be suppertime for them. We were next door to Bob's Big Boy—yeah, *that* Bob's Big Boy, where Drew Carey used to hang out all the time. Bob's Big Boy in Burbank is a great place for hanging and eating. Good burgers and spaghetti and real grilled cheese with the orange cheese and butter and white bread. We sat down, and the boys ordered all the above stuff.

The server came over, and I asked her for "A plain baked potato with nothing on it. Nothing. No oil on the outside, and no salt or pepper on it. No butter, chives, or sour cream—nothing. Just a plain potato."

"Really?" she asked.

"Yeah, really, thanks."

My buddies were shocked. "What's with the potato? Why you eating just a potato?"

They were my friends, so I owed them an explanation. "Fuck you, that's why."

That didn't shut them up, but who cares? They made some potato jokes, but even brilliant writers don't have a lot of potato material, so we went back to talking about the amazing projects we all had in mind that "The Man" was keeping us from doing. Here's the nutty part: they forgot about the potato, and more shockingly, so did I!

When the food was delivered, I coveted their salty greasy goodness, but after we all took our first bites, we just settled into eating and enjoying the company. After the first bite of anything, I don't really taste it anyway. Then it's just an activity. It's something to do with my hands while everyone is talking. I was so happy with my potato. I finished my potato and was still hungry, so I had another potato. Then I had another. We were all finished, and I felt great.

I'd prepared for this big potato test, and it was so easy. I felt great. Every other time I'd left that restaurant, I'd felt like shit. I'd always eaten too much and always felt terrible, sluggish, and a little sick. I'm not blaming Bob's—the food is prepared well, and it's fine food. It's not their fault that it took me until I was almost sixty years old to learn to feed myself properly.

DAY 12: 284.9

Back to Vegas. CrayRay and I had timed this just right, as my family was visiting Grandpa in the Caribbean. I had nothing to do but stay home, eat potatoes, sleep, take freezing showers, and do shows, and I even had a couple of days off from the show. It was time to be low-key and just let metabolic winter flow over me. Well, metabolic winter did flow over me, and I got a cold. I called CrayRay and told him I had a cold, that I was sniffling and felt like shit. I kind of expected him to say, "Well, you better have some orange juice and some chicken soup and a steak and get well and then start this again," but he didn't. He said, "Good; it's easier to take it easy and not eat when you have a cold. This is good."

Crazy fucker.

DAY 13: 285.8

I don't even know what happened in that couple of days. My family was gone; I was feeling shitty and ate nothing but potatoes and slept a lot. A real lot. I met Goudeau at a coffee place to drink coffee and talk about potatoes. I had a cold, but that wasn't a big deal. I get colds all the time. I do shows and scream like a nut and always end up exhausted, so I'm fighting a cold every six weeks or so. It's just stupid, and they last forever. But that cold I got during the potato famine . . . as of this writing, it's the last cold I've gotten until I was overworked on Broadway eight months later. Every eight months is better than every six weeks. I yell just as much. I work just as hard. I get just as tired. I'm around young children who go to school—but two colds in ten months.

I will not claim to you that the diet stopped me from getting colds. I have no control. I have no double blind. This isn't a scientific test. But I feel a lot better, and part of feeling a lot better is not getting sick. Maybe it's tied a bit to diet. I really don't know.

DAY 14: 284.0

Wow. Wow.

I'd lost about twenty pounds in fourteen days—but that wasn't the big news. As the weight dropped off me, CrayRay started laying the real info on me: fat wasn't the problem, fat was the symptom. I didn't start this diet because I wanted to be in the *Sports Illustrated* swimsuit edition, I started it because I wanted to get off the blood pressure drugs. The weight loss, the fat loss, was not the goal; it was a side effect. This day really showed why I needed to have a doctor involved. Every day I took my blood pressure and pulse with my

Withings blood pressure cuff, and that groovy little thing sent the info to both CrayRay and my doctor. We'll never know whether it was the weight loss, the lack of salt and other shit in my diet, or the magic healing power of potatoes, but my blood pressure was going down.

My pulse and BP were not just going down a little, they were going down faster than me on my high school girlfriend. On Day 14 my pulse hit 38. That's some really dangerous shit. When they talk about rapid weight loss being dangerous, this is what they mean. The very drugs that had kept me alive when I was living on salt and fat could now kill me. At around this time my blood pressure hit 132/64. That's not too low—it's still a little above normal—but for me to be on the high side of the normal range was astonishing. My doctor was talking to other doctors as well as to CrayRay, and they pulled me off one BP medication, and after a little more discussion they pulled me off another. I stopped taking two blood pressure drugs that I had been taking every day for years. This is stuff that can't be done alone. Even my doctor couldn't do it alone, and he's a great doctor. He needed advice and pulse checks and BP readouts all the time. It was like an emergency now to get me off the things that used to be keeping me alive. After just two weeks, I was off two meds. It seemed possible that this CrayRay shit was working.

Two weeks had flown by, and now I was "the potato guy." A friend of mine from a '90s punk band came backstage with his son after our show to hang out. I was very comfortable holding court, making jokes, and eating my baked potato. It felt so natural, even in front of a punk dad. Except for the continuing light-headedness during the show, I felt I could have kept up the potato famine forever, but CrayRay had other plans. It was time for Goudeau and me to have corn on the cob.

Goudeau and I would have corn! If you don't think that's a big fucking hairy deal, you haven't understood a word of this book.

PISS AND SPIT

Shockingly, I'm not a big fan of fart jokes. I just don't like them. When it comes to obscenity, I like sexual; I don't like scatological. I'm really comfortable talking about fucking and all that goes with it, but the fart and shit stuff—it just doesn't strike me as funny. I'm a dad, and my children are nine and ten years old, so there's a lot of fart humor and discussion, and I have been known to laugh along with them. I made *The Aristocrats*, and there were plenty of fart and shit jokes in that, but they were told in order to make an intellectual point. Or something.

When you're dealing with a profound diet change, when you take the human body down to a cup of beans a day, you're going to be dealing with issues that involve shit and farts. It's interesting to me that as the microbiome changes and the meat-eating critters in us die and the vegetable-eating critters have a party, the body adjusts and is really very comfortable with going to all vegetables. At least, that's what happened to me. It wasn't painful or embarrassing. The first few weeks were a little different, what with the, you know . . . farts and stuff, but it seemed to settle down after a while. If you don't think farts are funny, more than a cup of beans a day can be a challenge, but I made it through. It was surprising how fast my body adjusted to such a radical change in diet. My body adjusted before my sense of humor had to.

I guess I kind of expected that, but I was shocked by what happened to my piss and spit. I wrote earlier that I used to be on diuretics for my blood pressure, and it was hard to drive for even fifteen minutes to the airport in the morning without having to stop. When I was fat and sick, when I had to pee, I *really* had to pee. All of a sudden, I'd have to pee really badly. And I peed a lot. CrayRay says that peeing isn't about getting rid of the liquid in the bladder, it's about getting rid of the waste products from excess amino acids. When you eat a "protein-rich" (whatever that means) diet, the body has to get rid of a lot of amino acids, and it washes those away with piss. Add my former protein-rich diet to the diuretics I was taking, and it's a wonder I had any time to read, I was peeing so much.

As soon as I started eating nothing but potatoes, and later transitioned to the rest of the CrayRay diet, peeing was no longer an emergency. I would have to pee, but it felt like I had to pee within twenty minutes, not five. It was a lighter compulsion, more controllable. But I sure wasn't peeing less. The volume of the pee was greater, the length of time it took to pee much longer. It was, like, twice as long. And I was peeing clear liquid. All of a sudden I controlled my pee; it no longer controlled me. That wasn't one of the reasons I went on the diet, but it was a great side effect.

I also stopped drinking as much. The healthy thing I've always done was to drink enough water. I drink seltzer—carbonated water. I have those soda-making machines all over the place, and I have decaffeinated loose-leaf tea. Everyplace where I spend a lot of time—my office, our kitchen, my dressing room, backstage—I have machines keeping water carbonated and boiled at my fingertips. I love drinking water and tea. It's a nervous habit with me. It's entertainment, and it makes me feel good as well. On my Standard American Diet, I was thirsty all the time. I'd wake up and have two liters of seltzer and a big pot of tea, and then at least a liter of seltzer with every meal, with lots in between as well.

When I do the *Penn & Teller Show*, I talk a lot. Teller doesn't talk, so I'm talking for ninety-three minutes. There are bottles of water and tea all over the backstage area. Every time I exit the stage, one of our crew guys puts water in my hand. Occasionally I'd have to station a crew member just offstage so I could reach behind the curtains and grab some water while I was still onstage talking. We live and work mostly in Las Vegas, which is in the stinking desert, and it gets dry. There's a thing called "Vegas throat" (the medical condition, not Céline Dion's nickname), and you have to hydrate all the time.

At least, that was true on the Standard American Diet. Now that I'm on the CrayRay diet, I don't have to drink all the time. I still enjoy my seltzer and tea, but I never feel thirsty. Never. I guess the absence of massive amounts of salt and sugar, and the presence of all that water in the vegetables, means I just don't need to drink as much. I noticed right away, even during the two weeks of nothing but potatoes, that I didn't need to drink as much. Potatoes might seem pretty dry, but in reality they're little bags of water. My whole mouth changed. It feels cleaner and stays wetter. When I walk backstage during one of Teller's endless solo numbers, I don't reach for water right away; I can fix my hair and maybe blow my nose or ask our crew if there are any problems—but I don't need water or tea.

We end our ninety-three-minute show with the Bullet Catch, so after eighty-eight minutes of talking I catch a bullet in my mouth. I used to have to think of lemons to keep my mouth wet enough to stop me from gagging on the bullet in my teeth. But as soon as I got off the SAD diet, everything changed. My mouth was now so wet that I had to suck in air through my teeth to keep my mouth dry enough to drop the bullet into the volunteer's hand without drooling on him or her. That's a pretty big difference.

I pee more pure water than ever before, but never with desperate urgency. My mouth always feels clean and moist, even in the desert, and I'm rarely thirsty. I just drink water and tea for entertainment.

None of these side effects were advertised with CrayRay's diet, but I love them. I love the changes to my system.

Wow.

CORN IS CANDY

One of the basic rules of the CrayRay program is to take it really easy during the potato phase. Some people even cut out the potatoes and turn it into a fast, consuming nothing but water. But I was a weird case. I needed to actually eat potatoes during the potato phase, because I was doing shows every night, and that turned out to be more activity than CrayRay or I thought. I was running around, yelling, and thinking for a couple of hours a night. I would have liked to have done the first part of the diet as a potato vacation. When I think about going to some cabin in the mountains and eating potatoes, reading, napping, and fucking for two weeks, it seems pretty perfect, but I don't take vacations. Since my family was out of town, I could rest, nap, and watch the Three Stooges during the day, but I still had our show every night.

I was deep in CrayRay's metabolic winter, cramming down the

spuds and dozing, but I still had to get up and run around every night
in a bright summertime show. I wasn't really doing potato time right,
but still, it was getting results, and it wasn't that hard. It was more
extreme, crazier, and easier than any diet I had ever done.

The Monday before Christmas, Goudeau came over and we
hooked up the Sansaire. Corn was a big deal, so we were going to
make putting plain corn in boiling water as gourmet as we could.
I vacuum-sealed our corn (it took me four tries; I'm an idiot) and
dropped it into the perfect-temperature water, and we timed it to the
second on our phones. We could have just dropped the naked corn in
the pot and pulled it out after a while, but we dug the process.

Goudeau and I like to laugh. No one laughs easier than Goudeau.
Goudeau has a love of life that's inspiring. He's one of my cohosts on
Penn's Sunday School, and he giggles through the whole show. Some
asshole on Twitter said he's just a sycophant sucking my comedy dick,
and I guess you could feel that way if you never spent time with him
outside of the podcast. Goudeau giggles through our preshow prep,
he giggles through the postshow discussions, he giggles on the way
back to his car, and when you call him in the car, he answers with a
giggle. When he does his brilliant twelve-minute juggling show, he
giggles through the whole thing. Goudeau is one of my best friends,
and I've watched him go through some pretty bad times. I've seen
Goudeau cry, but I've never seen him far away from a giggle. I asked
him once why he giggled all the time, and he explained that when he
was a child, he didn't giggle. When Goudeau was a child, he snickered
all the time like a cartoon dog. His mom told him that snickering like
a cartoon dog all the time would hold him back in life, so she worked
with him to turn his snicker into a giggle, and this constant giggle is
where he landed. Why was he snickering all the time to begin with? A
better question is, why the fuck aren't we *all* snickering and giggling
all the time? We all know what life is; you can snicker like a cartoon

dog or you can weep like Leonard Cohen. I do both. Goudeau giggles.

When we took our first bite of corn, there was no weeping or giggling; there were belly laughs. It was shocking. It was nothing like any corn I'd ever tasted. It was sweet like candy. It was red-glossy-cracking-candy-apple-coating-at-the-fair sweet. It was maple-sugar-on-snow-in-New-England-with-my-sister sweet. It was baked-Alaska-and-sugar-straight-out-of-the-packet-at-a-diner-as-a-child sweet. And it wasn't just sweet, either. Those ears of corn had so many flavors. Those ears of corn were sweet like life. My favorite Bob Dylan line (and that's saying something) is "It frightens me, the awful truth of how sweet life can be." The corn was complicated-sweet like that line. Perfect sweet. Grown-up sweet. I-have-two-children-whom-I-love-and-I-don't-want-to-die sweet. Laugh-your-ass-off-with-your-buddy-Goudeau sweet. Two weeks of potatoes had knocked us out of our heads. We were out of our fucking crazy food-is-fat-sugar-salt dream world. Corn used to have no flavor at all for me. It was just fat and salt, because I'd always covered it in butter and salt. Corn tasted just like popcorn, and popcorn tasted just like lobster, and steak, and every other salty, fatty food, which was every food I ate. SAD had driven me out of my real-food-lovin' mind. I'm from Western Massachusetts, and I'd gone to farms to get corn that had been picked just an hour before. When my dad and I shucked it outside the house, the corn had the crisp sound and complicated smell of summer about to turn into fall, and then my mom would throw it into boiling water for an eyeblink, and the smell was perfect and complicated, and then . . . I smothered it with butter and salt. What the fucking fuck?

Now I was eating bullshit, supermarket lived-in-a-truck-for-a-week jive-ass corn, and all the sweetness of life was in every kernel. Months later, after I had lost my weight, our family visited Grandpa in Georgia, and he took us to one of those places where you pick the vegetables yourself and then leave money in a basket. It was raining, but who cares. Moxie ruined her little-girl shoes in the mud, but we still went. I didn't pick even one ear of corn or one tomato; I just stood in the rain watching my family carefully pick the corn and deliver it to me, and standing in the rain, looking at my children, my glasses covered with rain from the outside and tears from the inside, I ate that raw, naked love of life. I didn't need fucking butter or even a pot of water. When I saw *Last Tango in Paris*, Brando demonstrated the proper use of butter, and I just didn't get it at the time. Yeah, fresh-picked corn in the rain in Georgia, just picked by my son, laughing in the mud, is pretty great. But, you know, store-bought shitty corn in the middle of the desert with my snickering buddy is pretty good, too.

It's certainly an exaggeration to say that the potato famine taught me how to enjoy real food, but I don't know a way to tone it down and still make it read the way I mean. Goudeau and I had become giggling hippies saying "Wow" at plain corn.

Matt Donnelly, our coworker on *Penn's Sunday School*, started the CrayRay program several weeks after we had, and when he got to his Corn Day, he thought he was being punked. His first honest taste of corn was so sweet that he thought his wife had dipped it in a sugar solution just to fuck with him. He figured Goudeau and I put her up to it, and we all know Sarah well enough to know she'd do it. We hadn't and she didn't, but only because we didn't need to. Corn is crazy sweet on its own, as long as you haven't spent years beating your senses of taste, smell, and hunger with fat, sugar, and salt. We were ready to taste food in a whole new way.

I love dirt-dumb rock 'n' roll. I love three-chord rock 'n' roll: two guitars, bass, and drums behind a guy screaming about fucking. I love that. And that's what I listened to for a long time. It's easy music to listen to. You don't have to know much. You don't have to develop anything. You don't have to think; you just wiggle your ass and bang your head. It's great, easy music. If I'm in the middle of listening to

Chuck Berry's Golden Decade Volume 2 or "Bang Bang" and someone asks me if I want to stop and listen to a little *Wozzeck* by Alban Berg, well, Bang Bang outta the room, Alban, you know we don't want it. But for whatever reason, years ago, I got a little sated with four-on-the-floor and spent a little time learning and freshening my ears. I kind of started lyrically with Dylan and musically with Zappa, and then slid into some Varèse and Miles. I started to realize that music could be more than even the joy of rock. It took me years and years of Sun Ra, Stravinsky, Bach, Mingus, and Coltrane, but I changed. I still like rock 'n' roll, but . . . well, much less often. Eating the SAD is like being in a disco blaring three-chord four-on-the-floor music all day and all of the night. There might be a string quartet playing Bartók on the bandstand, but you'd never know it. I had been blaring those three chords—Fat, Sugar, and Salt—to the beat over all the complicated richness of the real food being drowned in butter.

Yeah, I lost the weight for my health. And yeah, I'm glad that I look better and fit better in my clothes. And I'm wicked glad my dick looks bigger. But putting all that aside, CrayRay also gave me an enjoyment of food that wasn't just da salt to da sweet to da fat to da beat and then to da repeat. Two weeks of potatoes. Two weeks of tasting plain food straight out of the dirt set me up to be able to taste the joyous excitement of plain corn. I was on my way to real enjoyment of real food, and that was making Goudeau and me laugh, because everything makes Goudeau and me laugh.

Those of you who know me know that there are few things I love more than an overextended metaphor, and I really want to keep this three-chord, fat/sugar/salt thing up for the whole book, but sometimes it seems backward to me. What if rock 'n' roll is plain corn and twelve-tone German opera is the fat/sugar/salt thing? Doesn't that also make metaphorical sense? Is blue cheese more like Schoenberg or the Troggs? But I think the metaphor is okay. I'm talking about our culture. I don't know what happens if you try this experiment on a child who's never heard Elvis or Bach. A child who's never had a carrot or a doughnut. But for me, the commercial stuff that plays to our simplest desires is rock 'n' roll and fat/sugar/salt. Rock 'n' roll can be complex—my favorite artist in any form is Bob Dylan, and my buddy chef Jet Tila can make fat/sugar/salt taste like *Blonde on Blonde*—but I still think the metaphor feels right. When I turned off pop radio, I found richer sounds; and when I stopped eating SAD all the time, I could taste bebop straight out of the ground.

All my tastes changed after those two weeks of potatoes. Foods that I used to not like or have much of an opinion about became my favorites. Every kind of mushroom had a different flavor, and each individual mushroom had slight differences. One batch of Brussels sprouts tasted different from another from the same store. Fruit had variety among species and individuals.

I have a very good friend whom I wrote about (in a very thinly disguised way) in my novel *Sock*. He's a carny buddy of mine who went nuts eating nothing but candy. He finally got down to eating only Jolly Ranchers. I talked to him about it a lot, as he was shaking and twitching in his trailer behind the Walmart where we had parked over a storm drain for unpleasant and illegal reasons. He said it had started to disgust him that he didn't know what he was going to bite into when he bit into an apple. Sometimes sweeter, sometimes mushier. He couldn't tell what he was going to get. Big Macs gave him constancy for a while, but he started to be able to tell one individual Big Mac from another, and the differences filled him with disgust. Candy bars had more consistency, but temperature could surprise him. He ended up with just Jolly Ranchers. Two watermelon-flavored Ranchers were closer to each other than any two pieces of real watermelon could ever be. When I think about his argument now it doesn't get crazier to me, it gets saner and saner. The more I think about it, the more I think my buddy is right. Pears are the worst. Pears will always fuck you. You get a nice ripe pear, sweet and firm, and you bite in and you think, "I'm going to eat nothing but pears for the rest of my life," and then the next one you bite into is mealy or hard or just . . . an asshole. Pears always fuck you in a way that a sour apple Jolly Rancher never will. You can trust a Jolly Rancher. You can't trust a pear.

Trust or variety? My mom and dad would take me on vacation road trips and we'd stop at Howard Johnson's instead of the local restaurant because they "didn't want to gamble." Type "Katy Perry" into the create-a-station-based-on-this-song-or-artist box on your computer, and you'll get really good, solid sour apple for the rest of your life. Type in "Sun Ra," and you have no idea what kind of mealy pear will be whaling on your dick. Consistency or adventure? Sour apple or real pear?

I was fifty-nine years old and I had eaten nothing but CrayRay potatoes for two weeks. I was ready for some variation in my diet. Our three reliably satisfactory chords, fat/sugar/salt, were gone for two weeks. I was ready. And when I started branching out slowly into nontubers, it was clear that everything had changed. I no longer had any idea what I liked. Let's talk about peppers. Not groovy, spicy peppers—they were part of the bad diet, and they're an even bigger part of the good diet. But bell peppers? I've always hated those fucks. I never liked the taste, and they made me belch, but that wasn't what I really hated about them. I hated their attitude. They're supposed to be a vegetable, but they feel exactly like the tip of your nose. Go ahead. Reach up and push on the tip of your nose. It feels fine for the tip of a nose, but it also feels just like a bell pepper. That ain't right.

Bell peppers are also hoity-toity assholes. They're not content to just be there for the eating, like a potato, or greens, or a carrot. I've always loved carrots. Carrots are about as trustworthy and humble as you can get in a vegetable. Bell peppers are fuckwads. The pepper has to break open with a weird sound. What the fuck is that? And you've got a whole lot of empty space in the middle of what's supposed to be a vegetable. Empty space and a few impossible-to-get-rid-of seeds. A carrot is all vegetable; how does a bell pepper get off with a big fucking air pocket in it? I'll take that kind of shit from a cantaloupe, but fuck you, bell pepper.

I still kind of feel that way about bell peppers; they still have a shitty attitude, but they taste okay to me now. I still won't feel them— fuck that, I'll feel my nose instead—but I'll eat them. Potatoes gave me that. I wouldn't know how much I'd really changed for months after that first ear of corn, but at the end of my potato weeks, I liked all foods. All the prejudice went away. I was knocked into free love.

Once in a while I'm going to go see Twisted Sister play some rock 'n' roll really loud, and once in a while I'm going to have a steak with Gorgonzola and a side of bacon mac and cheese, but most of the time, I'll be listening to Bach and eating a salad. That's what potatoes did for me.

Fuck, that corn was good.

FROM POTATOES TO
THE NEW YEAR

DAY 16: 284.0

The potato famine was over, and we'd had our first corn high that can never be matched.

From then on we would be eating nutrient-dense, calorie-deficient vegetable stews and taking a bunch of cold showers until we reached our target weight. I'd lost eighteen pounds in fourteen days of eating potatoes. I was a quarter of the way to my target weight after just two weeks. Wow. That's kind of nutty good. But the report from the scale was nothing compared to how I felt. Every moment of every day I felt great. I'd gotten through those couple of sluggish potato days, and since then I'd felt wonderful. I'd never felt like this on a diet before; I'd always felt deprived and like I was getting nothing out of it. I'd also felt guilty for not doing it quite right. Diets are like Christianity: they are set up so that you can never be sure you're doing everything right. It's your fault.

If I were a Catholic (if I were a Catholic, shoot me—but I have other points to make first) and I were sure that everlasting life lay in the balance, the entire talent list for kink.com couldn't get me to fuck outside of wedlock. Not even a blow job. I'm sure that if everlasting life and the pleasure of the lord almighty were at stake, I wouldn't even jack off. I believe I could follow even those insane antihuman rules perfectly. But religion is set up so that even perfect is never good enough. It's set up to fuck even the compulsive nuts. Religions have that coveting thang built in to take us down. Now, I say "set up," but I don't think there's any conspiracy. I don't believe, like many of my atheist siblings, that churches are run by people who make plans for how best to control others and then implement those plans for their own power and pleasure. Believing in a cabal of cardinals who create religions to dominate the masses seems a little too much like believing it wasn't Lee Harvey Oswald who popped Kennedy. Evil conspiracies are too much like god. We all have an urge to believe that someone bigger than us is in control, even if that someone is evil. It might be even more reassuring if that someone is evil; it would certainly explain all our troubles. But I don't believe in human puppeteers. I don't even believe in evil. The biggest insult I can give to Christianity is to say that I believe it evolved. Old religions that didn't have all this crazy-ass, manipulative, destructive, jive-ass shit simply fell away, and the ones that grabbed people by the ovaries and balls flourished. I'm such a hard-core atheist that I don't even believe churches were created. I think even they evolved. That's how atheist I am.

My buddy, mentor, hero, closest-thing-I-have-to-a-god James "Amazing" Randi explained that when you're sick, one of three things can happen: you can get better, you can get worse, or you can stay the same. As long as quacks can explain all of those three, they can stay in business. And that's not hard to do:

If you got better—this bullshit is working.

If you stayed the same—this bullshit stopped it from getting
worse.

If you got worse—we have to do more of this bullshit because it
takes time, and you're not doing it quite right; it's your fault;
be patient. Be my patient and keep buying my bullshit.

Diets always had enough wiggle room for me to worry that I
hadn't done something right, that I had cheated, and the lack of results was my own fault (which it was, for picking the wrong diet—
"You fucked up, you trusted us"). Diets always had those three quack
explanations covered. When I was counting calories, I had to estimate
what three ounces of tuna came to. I wondered whether that hamburger wasn't lean enough, or if the bun was too big. Could I have
gone a little heavier on the dumbbells? Was I really at the point of
exhaustion when I stopped? I always felt I was fucking up a little.
And when I wouldn't get the results I was promised, it was because I
had cheated a little. I went my whole fucking life without jacking off,
but I'm still full of sin because one of the MILFs had a nice ass and I
had carnal thoughts that I couldn't control well enough to please god.
That's how diets work.

I couldn't run CrayRay's system quite perfectly because it would
have meant not doing shows, but it still worked. There were a few
gray areas. I could eat all I wanted, but only of certain foods, and
only during what Ray referred to as the "fed window." He tells all the
"CroNuts" (Ray CROnise + "nut"—self-explanatory) to try to keep
the day's eating within a five-hour window while trying to lose weight,
and it's pretty useful and fun for maintaining, too. That means going
nineteen hours without food every day. Pretty black and white. I guess
maybe my cold showers weren't quite cold enough or I had a little too
much rice, but it was pretty clear that I was following the rules, and

when I didn't quite follow the rules . . . it still worked. It's the opposite of Christianity. Salvation without sin.

The weight was just melting away, and with it a lot of my free-floating food guilt. My friend and now fellow "CroNut" Matt Donnelly pointed out that guilt is a limited commodity. Feeling guilty every time you eat, whether you're on a diet that you're not doing quite right or you're just a fat fuck trying not to care, is a drain. Living in a state of constant guilt about eating is like being a Christian living in a constant state of guilt over fucking original sin. The difference is that the fat fucks go back to the Garden of Eatin' and eat all the forbidden fatty fruit over and over again themselves instead of every new generation being born in hate and pain, so it's kind of a wash. There's a lot in life to honestly feel guilty about. I should laugh at my wife's puns and try to enjoy her show tunes more. I should spend more time with my children, not snap at Teller, not write "Fuck you" on Twitter (I'm a little more guilty about being slightly proud of that, too). There's a lot of stuff to worry about without that fucking constant guilt that came with every mouthful when I was a fat fuck. And I'd coat that guilt with fat and wash it down with sugar water so I could swallow it easier.

I told Ray that one of the things I wanted out of his plan was the ability to read more of the newspaper in a detached way. I try to read the *New York Times* every single day, but sometimes I get too busy (and that's something else I feel guilty about). They print articles about health and the social effects of drinking, recreational drug use, and smoking. There are articles on domestic abuse and racism. Features on people gaming all sorts of financial and political systems for their own gain. Articles about all kinds of crime, anti-vaccers, spreaders of drug-resistant superbugs, and the proliferation of nuclear arms and other weapons of mass destruction. I read those with as much compassion as I can muster, but without any subjective worry. I don't smoke, I don't drink, I've never hit anyone in anger, I don't do B&E anymore, I don't have TB or Ebola, and I don't have any operational nuclear warheads—and it'll take me at least ten years to produce them unless you trust me to self-report my own personal inspections. For the most part, reading the news is a little cold and distant, and I like that.

But then there would be some sort of article about fat-fuck America. About the government deciding that they could stop diabetes by making people who buy soda give the government more money. An article on how diets don't work, but maybe if Michelle Obama had a nice garden, people wouldn't die as much from heart disease. I couldn't just read those articles and jump to the next one. I had to take time to blush as I read. I had to worry. I had to think about whether I wanted to finish the article and make myself feel worse or just skip to Krugman saying that if I don't agree with him on everything, it is my single-minded goal to destroy not only America's economy but also the whole world's security and economic safety. Krugman long ago forfeited his power to make me feel guilty, but the fat-fuck thing really made me crazy. It took guilt-energy to read those articles. No matter what they were writing about—BMI, "morbid obesity," "eating ourselves to death," "hypertension"—they were writing about Penn Jillette. I begged CrayRay to make it so reading about obesity was the same as reading about people who drop their genitals into hot blow-dryers: I wanted to think, "Hey, that *used* to be me!"

We started our new groove. CrayRay sent us recipes for new things to try. Although I have cooked on TV, I don't cook when there aren't cameras around, and my family wasn't in town, so Goudeau came over and cooked for the two of us. We had some black beans, rice, and corn, but I think we fucked it up. There was too much salt in the beans, but we ate them anyway (and didn't have to be forgiven for our sin). I had a couple of potatoes before the show, and goddamn it, I still got light-headed onstage. Fuck. After the show I had nothing to eat, not even a potato, because for the next few months we wanted to keep our fed window as small as possible.

I now think my hypertension and my obesity were caused by my constantly fed state. I was always eating. Eating well or eating badly, it didn't matter; I was always eating. My body never got a rest. I understood from CrayRay that one of the fastest ways to gain weight is to eat frequent small meals full of fat, and then exercise. It sure worked for me. When I'd finish eating, the "postprandial digestive process" (I got that phrase from CrayRay) was set in motion. It takes four to six hours to clear the blood of the rises in amino acids, lipids, and carbohydrates from food. If I drank alcohol, that would be in there, too, but I don't. Alcohol was the one thing I didn't have to quit, because I never started. The body has only three options for handling all this energy: it can store it, use it, or piss and shit it away.

Excess starch/sugar is stored as glycogen (whatever that is, but CrayRay *loves* this word) in liver or muscle tissue. I figured it was just turned into fat, but CrayRay says no. When I was eating frequently, my meals ended up being a big challenge to my body's effort to balance blood sugar; being constantly fed, my body had to get rid of all that glucose. This is why exercise feels great: because exercise burns mostly glycogen and not much fat. Exercise just made room for my next starchy/sugary meal to be stuffed away for later.

By restricting meals and dietary starch/glucose, we'd given my big old body a different problem than it had ever had in its whole fat-fuck life. After a couple of potato days, my body was still getting ready to groove on the next meal, but because of fucking CrayRay, all of a sudden it couldn't. Now my body was forced to balance glucose from my liver and use the fat from my reserves rather than from my mouth. This is a big deal. It had to get the energy to run my brain, manage blood glucose, and fuel my body from its reserves, which I had plenty

of and had never used. So when I first hit that low-calorie diet and ran
into the low-blood-sugar fog and wanted to just sit alone and watch
the Three Stooges, that was potato days three and four. That's when
most people quit this stupid shit and go back to eating all the time
and exercising like freaks.

Ray had forced us to be patient, and right after day four I started
feeling great. My body recognized that the doughnuts were no longer
streaming in and started to let go of all that stored glucose and fat.
Now I was eating Penn-fat burgers from inside my own body, with
extra Penn-fat mayo, and it felt great. As Joni Mitchell sang, "I'm sitting on my groceries." I was getting all the energy I needed from my
internal fat-pantry. All was going according to CrayRay's plan, except
for my still getting foggy during the show, and we had no idea how
to solve that. But for the most part, except for the most important
part of my day, my body was managing blood glucose levels with the
liver and not the mouth. It's supposed to be the liver that stops you
from feeling really hungry, and not the mouth. My whole life (and
your whole life, too, I bet), I'd been getting my energy directly from
my mouth. I was eating to regulate my blood sugar. But I was finally
teaching my liver to feed me. My liver takes the glycogen, feeds my
brain, and keeps my blood glucose balanced. It uses my fat the way it
evolved to be used. So there's no panic hunger from low blood sugar.

The last few paragraphs are just cut and pasted from CrayRay's
e-mails, blogs, and texts and then rewritten by me like a middle school
student copping the Wikipedia entry for Teddy Roosevelt and trying
to change just enough to not get busted. But I kinda sorta understand
it. At least, I think I do. The way I figure it, CrayRay wants us to be
playing the bagpipes and not blowing the sax. Even though I've never
played either—and I don't know whether you've played either, so I'm
breaking all my own rules of analogy—I still love this one. With bagpipes, you don't blow into that annoying, droning out-of-tune-flute

thing, you blow into the bag and then squeeze the air from the bag into the annoying, droning out-of-tune-flute thing. With the sax, you have to blow right into it for every note you want. I wanted to learn to eat like a bagpipe—to put the calories into storage and then let the liver blow them into my blood when it needed to keep me alive to write annoying, droning sentences like this one. Get it?

That's the way it works for animals and our ancestors. There's no eating constantly—life is feast and then famine. In many cases it really was a potato famine. One meal a day if you're lucky; two if you happen to win the hunter-gatherer lottery. Our food was always limited by what we could find and catch, not by our consciously cutting calories. How long have humans had too much food? Less than a century, and this is certainly not a worldwide phenomenon. For nearly all life on earth, the problem is too few calories—but for a few lucky assholes, the problem is too many. We're lucky until all the fat-sickness sets in. And it doesn't matter how many of us die from it; as long as we're dying after we've reproduced, evolution does fuck-all. Evolution works great to fix things that stop you from fucking in order to reproduce. Stuff that stops your heart from beating after you've reproduced can't be fixed. Evolution can't select for that. Evolution's sexy fuck hands are tied behind its back.

CrayRay forced my liver and muscle glycogen to do their thing while I kept my mouth shut. On day four, it was a pain in the ass, and then my lazy liver did its job and I was riding with king CrayRay. Use the mouth for fucking; the liver is driving. There would also be no exercise until I'd reached my target weight. Exercise is body-building; the body wants more food when you're exercising, and you can't possibly exercise enough to make up for the additional food you eat. We were forcing my liver to do the work, and giving my mouth and muscles a break. All the while, my fat was making up the difference and melting away.

During mealtime and for a few hours after (the fed window), energy needs are met primarily through the food just eaten. So that wasn't getting stored as fat. And as I ate fewer calories and ate them less often, my body spent more time each day in an early fasting state, during which it was using my stored fat for energy. So I wasn't starving at all—I was eating all the nice, marbled fat that was warehoused all over my body. I was eating the prime rib I'd been carrying around with me. I don't mean to spoil the ending, but over this period I dropped 0.9 pounds a day. A pound of fat is 3,500 calories, so I was burning 3,150 calories of stored fat every day. This isn't exactly true, because not every pound of that weight loss was fat, but it's pretty fucking close. I was pulling fat from everywhere. During this time my ring sizes ended up going from 13½ to 12½ and from 11½ to 9¾. Yup—I even had fat in my fingers. Now that I'm at my target weight, my card sleights are easier to do. Yeah—I have thinner fingers, and they're easier to sneak around behind a deck of cards. Amazing!

CrayRay called the post-potato phase we were entering "wait loss." It's a pun, because you don't exercise, you just wait, and the weight comes off. CrayRay would have us start eating vegetable dishes that would increase flavor intensities over the next month. We wouldn't get too much variety. He wanted to keep it a little boring. Food was not supposed to be entertainment. But after he'd slapped us down with that potato fortnight, we were happy with anything he'd give us. Get that liver working.

Goudeau was really really sick of potatoes, and most other Cro-Nuts hate them, but I liked them. I ate them more after the potato famine than I ever had before. I throw a little Tabasco on them, and they're great. They were my comfort food, and I always lost weight with them. But the upcoming months would still give me what I wanted: a plan for my eating that I didn't have to think about and couldn't fuck up. I had a few choices, but I ended up not using a lot of them. I like the same thing over and over. I like to just get eating out of the way.

DAY 22: 277.7

My wife, EZ, decided to start her own potato famine. She wasn't a fat fuck, but she felt that she'd feel better if she lost twenty-five pounds. She was thrilled by the physical, emotional, and mental changes the diet had brought to me, so she hounded CrayRay until he brought her on board. We wanted to have supper together at a restaurant, after which EZ would take the children to some stupid Chinese panda show and I'd leave to do my stupid show. This was our first family restaurant meal where I would be eating, and we were going to the Cheesecake Factory. EZ called ahead and told them I wanted three baked potatoes with *nothing* on them. Then she had to explain what she meant by "nothing." She had to say, "No salt or oil brushed on the skin—nothing." She also set up steamed asparagus and broccolini for me. EZ calling ahead made it really easy. I didn't have to be embarrassed by giving instructions to the server, and we let them know in advance I was going to eat a *lot*: three baked potatoes and three orders each of the vegetables.

This is one part of the CrayRay lifestyle change I hate: caring about what food I eat. I really hate it. It's not hard for me to give up the food, but it's really hard to give up the "I don't give a fuck" part of my personality. I've never been a picky eater, and I've always prided myself on that. I never had to order anything special in restaurants. I never had to ask anyone what was in anything or how it was prepared. I didn't care. I just ate it. I believe I'm still the only judge ever on *Iron Chef* who ate everything that was put in front of me. I ate the full serving of every food. I cleaned my plate. I ate the eyeballs out of the fish. Calvin Trillin taught me how to get the best food in any restaurant. He took me to Sylvia's, the soul food restaurant in Harlem, and he ordered for us. "Bring us anything you think we should try." Over the years I changed that to, "Bring us whatever you want, whatever you're trying to get rid of, whatever is going bad." I still do that with other things. When buying show tickets, I say, "Give me the seats you're trying to get rid of. Make your chart easier to sell to other people." I figure I do as well that way as I would by being a pain in the ass. Maybe better; but if I don't do better, I don't care. If it's a good show, properly directed, it's directed for every seat. If it's a good restaurant, all their food will be good. I'd order that way whenever I was with friends who would eat anything. My wife has always been a very picky eater, and that's part of the reason she was never a fat fuck. She cares what's in everything and tells the server how to tell the chef to cook the food—what griddle to use and how much butter and extra cilantro and a little fresh lime juice, please. I always find it a little uncomfortable, but she gets the food the way she wants it and she stays healthy and slim. She wins.

My buddies Tim Jenison (*Tim's Vermeer*) and Farley Ziegler (producer of *Tim's Vermeer*) and I were over in England working on a movie (*Tim's Vermeer*). All of us would eat anything (and yet Farley is slim and healthy; hmmm—maybe this whole book is bullshit), and when the three of us went out to eat together, we got the best meals ever. We'd go into fancy Indian restaurants and say, "Bring us whatever you want, whatever you're trying to get rid of, whatever is going bad," and we would get feasts. They told us what they were serving us, but I don't hear well and don't decode accents well, especially when the accent being attempted is English . . . so I had no idea. I just knew it was interesting and delicious. I've even tried, "Give me whatever is going bad" at chains like Chevys, and the couple of times I did it, it worked out great. I got stuff that wasn't on the menu, stuff the chef whipped up just for me, like she might make for her family. It was delicious.

I loved ordering like that. And if I wasn't writing a book on how my SAD diet was fucking killing me, that would be my advice on eating. We sometimes do private corporate shows, and the buyer will pay us a shit-ton of money and then tell me what "in" jokes to do and which tricks they want from our show, in what order, and who we should use for our audience "volunteers." The long-suffering Glenn tells them they'll get a better show if they let us make all those decisions, which is true, and they usually understand that. But if they insist, we give them what they ask for, and they're happy with that, too . . . but we know we weren't as good as we could have been if they had just let us do our jobs. I feel that way about everyone. I'm buying your expertise; I want you to do what you do. Whether it's Picasso or the chef at Chevys—do that thang you do, please.

CrayRay had taken away that announcing of my confidence in other people doing their jobs well. Less-fat-fuck-Penn was calling in advance, or, like the coward he is, having his wife call in advance to tell them, "He'd like three baked potatoes with nothing on them— no butter or sour cream or bacon bits, but also not even a brush of oil on the skin to make it crispy and properly brown; not even a few grains of kosher salt to give it a twinkle and some flavor. Nothing. And the vegetables should be steamed plain. Just plain. No oil, no butter, just plain—and three big orders of each, please." Soon we would add to that, "And a salad with no animal products and no grains at all. That means no cheese of any kind and no croutons— just vegetables with nothing on them. Nothing. No dressing at all. Some plain vinegar on the side, but nothing on the salad." It takes all the joy out of preparing food for me, but maybe my heart won't blow up this year.

"Listen, Mr. Picasso, my husband would like a painting, but it's very important there be no shapes and no colors in that painting at all. Understand? Just to be clear, he'd like flat white paint on canvas—no gloss, and, please, no brushstrokes—just plain flat white evenly brushed on the canvas with no texture. Thanks so much."

The Cheesecake Factory did a great job with my picky supper. It was the first time I'd had steamed asparagus since potato time. It tasted amazing. There were all these flavors that I'd never tasted before. I guess they must have always been there beneath all the hollandaise, but you couldn't prove it by me. I asked if I could have even more. I was within my fed window, so I could have all I wanted.

The children were eating what children eat at the Cheesecake Factory (getting them to eat better is a project we didn't want to tackle until we had me totally under control). I kissed them good-bye and went over to do the show.

I had eaten a lot, but I was still light-headed during the show, and during the worst part of the show. I was light-headed during the finale. We end our Vegas show with the Bullet Catch, and it's irresponsible of me to be light-headed during that. My diet was saving my life but fucking Teller.

Our version of the Bullet Catch is very safe. We, like Houdini, will not do anything more dangerous than sitting in our living rooms. Having a daily breakfast of eggs and toast with butter was more dangerous to me than doing our finale every night. We have layers and layers of protection, even though we use real guns and real shattered glass. People are coming to our show to laugh at danger and enjoy the excitement, and even if we didn't care about our own well-being, we should care enough about our audience's morality to not put ourselves in jeopardy while they're enjoying a show. My being light-headed onstage did not increase Teller's risk of having his head blown off, but it did increase his risk of being part of a show that sucked. If I skip a joke, the show is less funny. If I miss a move, the show is less deceptive. And if I'm spacey, the show is less crisp. All those things are bad and unfair to Teller.

If I had a different job and got a little light-headed, I'd just have to sit down for a second, or simply pause in my speech. In our show, I can't really do that. Where I'm standing, how I'm standing, what I'm saying, and when I'm saying it are all part of the show. Losing weight and feeling better were important, but I had to find a way to do it while not breaking my promises to Teller, our coworkers, and the audience.

DAY 25: 272.8

Day 25 was what others call New Year's Eve. New Year's is a big day in our family. We don't have any celebration on Christmas, so we save it for New Year's Day. That's when we exchange gifts. It's nice to be later than the other children, because we get to see what our children's friends got and which of those things our children liked the best; I suppose that, in principle, we should be able to benefit from stores marking down their plastic shit, but I think we just buy the children a lot of plastic shit to show them that their parents are better than Santa and Christ put together.

And New Year's Eve is a big deal for all our friends. Teller and I decided that to celebrate our success, we would take New Year's Eve off. That's unheard of in showbiz, but we do it. We don't like to end our year on a drunk audience, and we don't like driving with drunks. EZ and I have a little shindig at our house, and all our friends who don't want to get drunk come by and eat. CrayRay had decided that I could now have salads. This was a big hairy deal, because now there would be the taste of fruit. The most sweetness I'd had. I'd lost thirty pounds in twenty-five days. I was illin' and chillin' like little Bobby Dylan, but I knew New Year's Eve was going to be tough, tough, tough. We have all our friends over to not get drunk on New Year's Eve, and unfortunately, it's hard enough to find dozens of people who don't drink on New Year's Eve without also trying to insist that they don't eat, so we have plenty of food for them. EZ had planned "Happanini New Year," and she had all this great stuff for people to put together their own paninis. Roast beef, salami, all kinds of cheese and vegetables, and great bread. Oh dear. Everyone eating great sandwiches and chips and desserts and everything; just beautiful. I could have eaten vegetables, which would have given me some wiggle room, but I wanted to be hard-core. If there was one little crack in my willpower, I'd be cramming down handfuls of roast beef. I wanted to be perfect.

Although CrayRay allows it, I gave up caffeine long ago. I don't want recreational drugs to be part of my life. I don't like to time things. We had a great espresso machine with little decaf pods. I drank those like crazy. It kept my mouth bitter and my spirits up. One thing this diet taught me was to have a love for bitter. I dig it now. My drink of choice at Bucky's (and keep this in mind if you see me there and want to be kind) is a venti (it means "twenty") *decaffeinated* Americano with two extra shots. All the bitter and none of the speed. As bitter and blue as a jazz musician at 3:00 a.m. In the Vegas summer I sometimes have it iced.

On New Year's Eve, I just kept making and drinking little cups of espresso. I had two big CrayRay salads that EZ made for me with sweet dressing and new flavors, and then went back to espresso. At midnight, bringing in a new year in which I would be thinner, I celebrated by having a nice big tasty slice of . . . nothing, motherfucker. I was *doing* this thang.

It was made a little easier by people starting to really see the change in me. Thirty pounds ain't nothing. My clothes fit differently and my face looked different. We watched the Vegas fireworks from the roof of our house with the gang, and I felt cold and hungry going into the new year. Just the way CrayRay wanted me.

FROM NEW YEAR'S
DAY TO HALFWAY

DAY 26: 272.9

We Jillettes start our year running through the full range of human emotions in the first few hours. Every New Year's Day, before the presents, I buy a bunch of helium balloons at the nearby supermarket, and as a family we let them go in memory of all the people we love who have died. I started this tradition in honor of my mom, who died on the first day of 2000 after asking me to release the balloons that were in her room. The children join EZ and me in that sadness, and then we share the joy of presents and celebration. I added yet another new feeling in 2015. That was the first year I've awakened to a new year without feeling shitty from overeating like a freak the night before. I've never woken up hungover, of course, but I would still feel pretty shitty. I woke up this new year feeling great. I cried a little with my children as we watched the balloons disappear into the sky, and then laughed a lot over the presents. I felt great. I didn't need to eat anything until suppertime, right before the show.

For EZ, the new year started with two weeks of just potatoes. You would think that eating only potatoes for two weeks would be so miserable that if you watched someone go through it, you'd never want to do it. But EZ had watched most of my potato famine and couldn't wait to do it. She'd seen my new energy, my new joy, and my new looks. She couldn't wait to get on the potato train. But she found eating nothing but potatoes to be less fun than she'd thought. She was in a shitty mood. I had moved on to big salads, and EZ made them for me. That's how much of a trouper she is. I discovered that this diet even changed how long it took me to eat. I'd been able to bang down a double cheeseburger, fries, and a shake in less than ten minutes, but these salads were just so much more food, so many more mouthfuls. I was eating a whole family-sized bowlful of salad, dressed with only vinegar, all by myself. I'd start eating before the children even sat down to supper, and I'd still be eating when they were back at their homework. It sometimes took me forty-five minutes to eat my salad, and I shovel fast. I had cut my calories drastically, but I sure hadn't cut volume. I say I cut calories, because I know I did, but there was no calorie counting. I ate until I was full, eating just what CrayRay told me to eat, and didn't eat again until the next day.

DAY 30: 268.6

I went to see a magic show on my day off. My date was Piff the Magic Dragon. It was a really shitty magic show, and that's why Piff wanted me to go with him. It was a weekday right after the new year in Vegas, so the casinos were empty. Piff and I made the mistake we always make: we thought seeing a shitty show would make us laugh and feel superior. But it only made us sad and want to quit showbiz. I can no longer find joy in bad art.

We made a quick trip to a magic shop, and then Piff wanted supper. Remember that CrayRay didn't want me talking about my diet, so I just asked Piff where he wanted to eat. He wanted English food, so we went to an English pub called the Crown & Anchor here in Vegas. I thought I'd be able to find something to eat, but there was no baked potato, no rice, no plain vegetables. It was a real English pub. There was nothing acceptable for me to eat. If I'd been performing that day, it would have been a problem, but I didn't have to worry about being light-headed, so I ate nothing. According to CrayRay, eating nothing is the option that's most often overlooked. You get into a groove with your diet, and then you go out to eat with friends and there's nothing that's right for you on the menu, so you get something "close." "Well, they don't have plain salad with vinegar, so I guess I'll have a double cheeseburger and make sure I get it with lettuce and tomato so I'm kind of having a salad." I've thought that way. But there's always the option of eating nothing. One of the most important things CrayRay taught me was that there's no nutrient the human body needs every day. You need air every couple of minutes and water every couple of days, but there's no particular food you need to stay alive. At any given moment, I'm still weeks away from scurvy. The whole idea of "I haven't eaten anything today" being a bad thing had to go away, and that was a good thing. I just drank seltzer. It was awkward for about fifteen seconds. "There's nothing here I feel like eating, but I'm fine." Piff ate and I watched him, and who cares? In the end, I went more than twenty-four hours without eating and felt great. Just great. Crazy good.

Piff didn't want English dessert, but he wanted dessert, so I suggested Krispy Kreme doughnuts. I kinda wanted to show off to myself. I wanted to go to my favorite hot doughnut place and just have a cup of decaffeinated coffee. Kind of like Gandhi sleeping between two naked women to prove he could be celibate (or maybe because it's fun to sleep between two naked women). I didn't eat any doughnuts, but I sure enjoyed the smell (*exactly* like Gandhi and the women). Piff then decided to take me to the greatest, and weirdest, place on earth.

We went to a place called Café Teaze. It serves those weird Japanese bubble teas, like sugar water with tapioca floating in it, except that they're served by young women in lingerie. It's real lingerie, not showbiz lingerie, so from certain angles it's just a nude club. It's not lit like a strip club, it's lit like a place that serves weird bubble tea, so it's bright, bright, bright. It's the kind of light you rarely see lingerie in, even in the mirror in your own home. It's also cold, like stupid Vegas air-conditioning show-off cold. You're thinking hard nipples, and that's certainly part of it, but that particular feature is accompanied by all the women shivering: come for the erect nipples, stay for the hypothermia. This is heaven for CrayRay, with his crazy cold experiments. Shivering nearly naked women serving bubble tea.

That's weird enough, but the economics make it even weirder. The tea isn't overpriced, and there is no stupid high tipping (except from the Magic Dragon and me). So the women are walking around almost nude for less money than they'd make at a Starbucks, with less clothing than they'd wear at a strip club. Weird.

Who goes to a place like this? When we were there, a bit before midnight on a weeknight, it seemed like the clientele consisted of high school girls playing board games. Tables of young women with backpacks playing checkers and Monopoly. There weren't any creepy old guys other than me and my Magic Dragon.

We noticed there were no crosses around anywhere, so we figured the servers were most likely vampires who were not concerned about money or cold, just with finding new victims. That's where Occam's razor pointed us. I can't speak for my magic dragon, but I was fine with being bitten on the neck at midnight by a shivering, nearly naked Asian woman. That's as good a way as any to become undead.

DAY 31: 270.5

Skipping that meal with Piff and drinking water instead of vampire bubble tea meant that I'd gone twenty-five hours without eating. CrayRay loves this. Mini-fasts really make the liver work. I didn't have a show, so not only did I not worry about getting light-headed, I didn't actually get light-headed. I was sitting down more and yelling like a freak while running around less. I felt great.

Moxie was in cheerleading class (it lasted only two weeks, because god is kind), and I was helping Z with his arithmetic at a Mexican restaurant. He had some nachos and I had a few potatoes and a couple of tomatoes to get me ready for the day's show. CrayRay was still working to resolve my light-headedness. We decided to try an experiment. That night during the show, while Teller was onstage making a red ball dance around like magic (well, like magic with a thread attached), I ate a few glucose tablets backstage—the kind that diabetics use when their blood sugar is low. I continued to do that every night during the show for the rest of the diet phase, and I guess it kinda sorta helped. I didn't feel like I was going to faint, but I still felt kind of too happy to do the show. I was so energetic and full of life as the weight fell off me that my mind would wander and wonder during the show. *The Penn & Teller Show* is composed and memorized. We're doing tricks that look like miracles. We're doing tricks that look really dangerous. I can't just say whatever pops into my head. I have lots of other opportunities to improvise and ad-lib. I do the *Penn's Sunday School* podcast every week, and although I have notes, I'm really just talking and letting the conversation go where it wants. I can't do that in the live show; with rare exceptions, I have to stick to the script. Teller and the crew have to know where we are and what we're doing. My part is often to be the anchor that my coworkers cue off. That's not a hardship. I love planning the dive and diving the plan. I love trying to get the nuances a little better every night. I can do the show on autopilot; my mind can wander, and I can still do the show. And I think sometimes when I'm not "present," the show is even better. I've watched carnies perform on the bally with not even the slightest idea what the words mean anymore. Just pure rote recitation, and there can be so much beauty in that. Actors always talk about "being in the moment," but I'm not sure that performers are any different. But with the new diet, I wasn't going on autopilot. I was taking the controls too often. I was thinking too fast for the memorized lines. I needed glucose and a lot of willpower to do a show that was fast, funny, and amazing, but still not as fast, funny, and amazing as I was really feeling. I was getting to be like Steven Wright and had to get myself down for the show.

DAY 32: 268.3

DAY 35: 266.7

CrayRay let me add Tabasco. Hey now! Tabasco has some salt, but it has much less than many other hot sauces, and CrayRay thought it was okay. Now the whole world changed. The diet had been easy before, but now it was just full of joy. The amount of Tabasco that I can eat is astonishing. And with Tabasco, I can eat anything. Beans become chili. There are these little room-service bottles of Tabasco that I now keep in my pocket at all times. It means that at an airport, I can get a plain baked potato or some plain rice (Chinese fast food is better than Japanese fast food for this—the sushi places often add sugar and salt to rice, but Chinese places figure that since what they're going to put on the rice is all sugar, fat, and salt, they're okay leaving the rice plain) and just pour the Tabasco on. I love it. We have bottles everywhere—at the house, at the theater, in the car, in my pocket. I love it.

L.A. has the only vegan restaurant I've found where I can eat. It's called Real Food Daily. I'll write later about why I hate vegan restaurants—and a lot of stuff on RFD's menu falls under that rubric—but they've got one thing that's perfect: the "Real Food Meal." It's brown rice, beans, daily greens, land and sea vegetables, pressed salad, and a choice of one dressing or sauce. I get a little bit of peanut sauce on the side and eat just a couple of drops. This is a big bowl of food. Just a huge bowl. And when I was there I had two of them. I had two huge bowls of food. It's just so good and so filling. I didn't use the peanut sauce, but I sprinkled some Tabasco over eveything. I was very happy with my two bowls of food, and when I ended up back in Vegas, my scale agreed, too. "Withings," "Tabasco," "Real Food Daily"—with all these brand names, maybe I'm getting to be as good a writer as Stephen King.

While I was in L.A., I wanted to visit my buddy Andy, who was in the ICU for being a fat fuck, but I wasn't a family member, nor were we married, so I couldn't get in. It would take me a few months, but I eventually got him on the diet, and today he's down fifty pounds and feeling great.

You might assume that the reason I went to L.A. was to visit the friend who came close to death, but that would mean you don't understand my priorities very well. The reason I went to L.A. was to do magic for a dog. More precisely, Teller did magic for a dog, and I did the voice of the dog's interior monologue. The CW was doing some sort of awards show for dogs (find a need and fill it), and since our show *Penn & Teller: Fool Us* was going to air on the CW, we wanted to get some exposure. So there I was, rehearsing magic for a dog. Teller was doing sleight of hand with steak. I don't like dogs. Our family is a reptile family. Mox is allergic to dogs, and I'm creeped out by things being eugenically bred to look like our children and suck up to us, so Mox has geckos and Z has a bearded dragon. These animals were not bred to suck up. They don't even care that we're around. That's what I like in a domestic animal. We're a turtle, fish, and lizard family. We have crickets mailed directly to us, and our pets' supper sings to us. We like that.

We learned that dogs will not walk across a big, very well-lit, glossy floor. That's another reason an awards show for dogs is against nature. My friend was in the ICU, and I was watching my business partner do the French Drop with a ball of meat to fool a dog that was almost as big as me. We kept getting bigger and bigger dogs to do the trick for. I was losing weight so quickly and the dogs were getting bigger, so if we'd done this gig a few months later, the dog I'd be voicing would have been bigger than me. I was still a Newfoundland, but I was heading toward Shih Tzu.

Meanwhile, another dear friend of mine, Tony, was having open heart surgery in Chicago for being a fat fuck. Motherfucker; I think I made the right choice.

DAY 36: 264.9

I'm *OVERWEIGHT*! No longer obese. My BMI is 29. That puts me at the top of the overweight category. It's the first time in years that I haven't been obese. That's a big step. On *Penn & Teller: Bullshit!*, we did a big hunk on how BMI was total bullshit. The plan was always to do a *Bullshit of Bullshit!* show, in which we'd tear ourselves apart like we did all the other assholes and point out where we were wrong. But we were kind of right on BMI; it is bullshit. It's not a good way to judge health, level of fat, or weight. It's total jive, but even so, I kept checking it and was thrilled to finally make "overweight." That doesn't say anything about BMI—it's still just as bullshit—but it does say a lot about me: shallow, hypocritical, self-serving, lacking convictions and a moral compass (all true), but also no longer obese. The *New York Times* theater reviews are all bullshit, too . . . but they gave us raves on our Broadway show, and we celebrated that. Nothing here to be proud of—except no longer being obese, and having a well-reviewed show on Broadway.

I wasn't quite halfway through the program and I'd really hit a groove. I had my contrast showers every morning, and then I'd have one meal a day. Right before the show I'd have some sort of chili over potatoes, and that would get me through nicely, with the aid of a couple of glucose tablets. I was still light-headed now and again, but it wasn't too irresponsible for a guy who was just overweight. I was losing weight really fast and feeling better every day.

DAY 37: 264.3

I was five weeks into the cult, and I'd lost forty pounds. I had an interview with CBS for some jive thing, and everyone was scrambling around trying to find clothes that would kinda sorta look okay on me. I did the interview with safety pins running up and down my back gathering up what was now extra fabric. My jeans used to be tight at a 44 waist, and now I was loose in a 38, but I didn't want to buy many new pairs, because I wasn't going to be at 38 for long.

DAY 38: 264.8

I went to visit Moxie for lunch at school, and the servers noticed I was a lot thinner. It's getting to be the only thing anyone ever talks to me about.

Just chili every day, one meal a day, sometimes on rice, sometimes on potatoes. The potatoes and rice aren't really part of CrayRay's plan, but I seem to need them to be able to focus during the show.

My mom used to cut up radishes and cucumbers and put them in a bowl with apple cider vinegar and a little sugar, salt, and pepper. It's one of my favorite tastes of summer. EZ made it for me just like Mom did, but without the salt and sugar. Wow. Just so good. We bought an assortment of fancy-ass vinegars, all sorts of balsamics and some with, like, plum flavor, but you know, plain old apple cider vinegar is the best. I could drink that stuff straight, and not just because it would be a blasphemous travesty of holy communion but also because it's good for me and tastes great.

One of the downsides of this diet is that if someone looks at our pantry, it's pretty clear that at least one hippie lives here, and maybe a whole family of hippies. It's pretty disgusting. Although "organic" is bullshit and "no GMO" is bullshit, a lot of the food we buy is labeled that way. Now we have apple cider vinegar "with the mother." I use the cloudy vinegar that has cellulose mixed with the cooties that make apple juice into vinegar. I'm eating active cooties on my salad. It's just stupid. But I feel great and it tastes great and I'm losing weight.

Come hear Uncle John's Band.

DAY 39: 265.9

I've written a lot about the changes in my health and looks, but there were other changes going on. I was getting happier, even though this was a time of very heavy stress. Whenever I mention "work" or "stress," I don't really mean it. Viktor Frankl, in his essay about being a prisoner at Auschwitz, draws an analogy between suffering and gas, in that they both fill up whatever space they're put into. He says suffering completely fills the consciousness and soul, whether the suffering is great or small. This man, who lived through the worst suffering any humans have ever endured, says suffering is absolutely relative. I guess that's true for all people who suffer, but I'm in showbiz, so I don't suffer. I get annoyed and pissed off, and those things are not noble gasses. That's not suffering.

Please understand that anything I complain about is done with the full and constant knowledge that I have nothing to complain about. But I want to make a point about this diet: in my stress-free life, the time I spent on this diet was pretty stressful. I was working on a movie, and the people who were most important to me on the movie weren't getting along, and I was in the middle of it. My schedule was insane—flying all over the country, "working" from early in the morning to late at night. I had a lot of people tugging on my coat about everything. I've always considered myself a very happy person, but looking back on myself as a fat fuck, I wasn't that happy. I told myself I was happy and I tried to act happy, but I failed. There was a lot of quiet sulking as my two atoms of suffering gas bounced around, filling my nonexistent soul.

I'd lost over forty pounds, and I was backstage at a shindig in a big hotel ballroom full of TV critics. Teller and I were going to go out and announce that our new TV show would be coming out the next season, and then do a Q&A about it. I was being briefed by one of the suits on what I was supposed to say, and more important, what I was supposed to *not* say when I got out in front of the reporters. Now, my answer to a suit giving me that kind of briefing has always been, "Thanks and go fuck yourself, I'll say what I want." And that's exactly what I said . . . but now, being forty pounds lighter, I was smiling. I didn't mean it. It was a big change for me.

After that, one of the people I work closely with decided to sit me down and explain in detail how I'd recently fucked up a deal with a TV network. How our meeting with the suits had gone badly, and it was all my fault. He told me this at regular intervals, I think, to make sure I remembered that it wasn't his fault, and if I did as much for my career as he did for my career, he would be doing a lot better than the great he was doing. I think he's right. I did fuck up a meeting, and badly. I wasn't rude, I was just stupid. I am a Vegas comedy magician, and I was always trying to get some serious drama on the air with me as creator and writer. The meeting at Morton's had gone well (we'll see), but I fucked up meetings before that. And now it was time to remind me of that again while I sat backstage and got ready to go out and not lie like I was supposed to in front of the press. Normally that much hot suffering gas in the room would have bummed me out for a couple of hours, and I probably would have fucked up the press conference because I was bummed about fucking up an earlier meeting in the same way. But things had changed. I was a different guy. Along with the forty pounds I'd also lost a great deal of sadness and anger. I sat there while my failings were explained to me and "shuffled" (I wasn't really shuffling, I was working on a new false shuffle) a deck of cards and "listened" (I wasn't really listening, I was working on a new skinny false listen).

There's a lyric written by NRBQ, a wonderful band who put words to the Rebels' "Wild Weekend." It's one of the best descriptions of joy I've ever heard. Joey Spampinato sings, "The girl's a drag, but it don't even faze me." The things that were being said to me—"You're a fuck-up" and "Go onstage and lie about your show"—were certainly a drag, but it didn't faze me. I "shuffled" and "listened" and went on with my day. As it turned out, I did everything the suit wanted me to, and the conference went great. I think a lot of it was the weight loss. I've always been happy around my children, but now I was clearly happier. I was nicer to Teller. Now, when I say "nicer to Teller," that kind of makes it seem like I *was* nice to Teller, and now I was even more nice. I've never been nice to Teller. We're coworkers, at best polite and at worst rude to each other. I'm worse to Teller than he is to me, but now I was smiling at him more. I was happy to see him.

I have a very easy and pleasant life, and losing the weight made it more pleasant. In case I haven't mentioned this before, I'm an atheist. I do not believe there is any mind/body separation. All we are is our brains. We are chemical reactions. We are stuff. I haven't even really entertained the thought of a soul or even a mind for years and years, and yet I was beginning to see that wasn't true. This diet had shown me that I was depressed because I was a fat fuck. Not depressed because I wasn't good-looking or couldn't do certain things, or even because I was dying, but depressed because I was physically fat. There was something purely chemical that made me sadder. It's not that amazing, right? You're going to feel like you have less energy if you're fat and have to lug around all that weight, so why wouldn't that also be true emotionally?

I've written elsewhere about CrayRay taking me up in the vomit comet to get me weightless and how I stripped naked, sang "Barbarella," and threw up all over him. The way you achieve weightlessness is that the plane does parabolas. It flies straight up and then straight down in a sine wave. All the chatter afterward is about the glorious feeling of weightlessness and the giggly fun and the euphoria, but because it's a pretty equal wave, the up feeling of weightlessness (which is the airplane going down) is balanced by the down feeling of being twice your weight (which is the airplane going up). So, when I took that flight, I weighed about two hundred fifty pounds and experienced weighing almost nothing and weighing about five hundred pounds. The exact time changed with every parabola, but it was about thirty seconds in each state. And we did it over twenty times. There was a lot about this experience that was mind blowing, but the part that seems so relevant here is the mood changes. When I was weightless I was giggling, full of energy, and in love with life, and when I was five hundred pounds I was so sad and depressed I would almost cry. The airplane and my changes in weight caused these huge mood changes. Now I was seeing it in slo-mo. I didn't lose five hundred pounds in thirty seconds, but I'd lost forty pounds in about the same number of days, and I was happier. I was just plain motherfucking happier. And I'd started out pretty fucking happy.

DAY 42: 261.2

In the afternoon I went out with my family and a couple other families to the *Titanic* exhibit at the Luxor. It's just shit from the *Titanic*, but it's a nice exhibit and makes you very pensive. Tragedy can be relaxing. In the first room, our family was making too much noise. This guy came over and reprimanded EZ for "not being respectful" to the people who were trying to listen to the audio wands. She argued back, and I went over and got into it.

This was a change, I think because of the weight loss. When I was younger, the world was performance art, but as I've gotten older and more successful I tend to save my whimsy for when I'm "working." I've been very reserved in public—polite, respectful, and quiet. Some of that restraint must have been stored in some of the fat I lost. I decided to be crazy there in the *Titanic* exhibit, just for fun. The aggrieved guy told me to be respectful, and I said, "I haven't made a sound; what are you blaming me for?" He pointed to the group we were with, and to EZ. I said, "What? I don't know her. I'm not with them. Why are you talking to me?" He didn't know what to say (because he was dealing with a crazy person). I said, quietly and with great respect for all the people who had died on the *Titanic*, and for those who had bought the audio wands to hear about them, "Let's get her! Let's kick her ass. C'mon! Let's really fuck her up. Let's show her what respect means. Let's get her. C'mon, let's kick her ass." It made what had been an awkward and embarrassing situation insane. I like insane a lot more than awkward. Now it was performance art. He was completely in the right, and our family pulled it together after his reprimand. See? This is what happens when I'm in a good and energetic mood. I'm a different kind of asshole.

My wife was so pleased that I stuck up for her. It takes a special kind of woman to love me.

YOU SAY "PROTEIN,"
I SAY "FUCK YOU!"

"Are you getting enough protein?"

"Fuck you!"

"Are you eating nuts for your protein?"

"Fuck you!"

"You need to have some *meat, right—you know, for protein?"*

"Fuck you!"

"Aren't you weak without protein?"

"Fuck you!"

"How about some protein on your salad?"

"Fuck you!"

"Don't you have to eat really carefully and expensively to get the protein you need without dairy?"

"Fuck you!"

Hey, protein: go fuck yourself! No kidding, protein; fuck you.

I think the thing that made me fattest and sickest was worrying about getting enough protein. I "knew" I needed a lot of protein every day to be healthy, but I didn't really know what "protein" was. I just knew it was chicken and steak and cheese and fish and milk and pizza and peanut butter, and I needed a lot of it. I didn't just need protein every day, I needed it every few hours. I kept little packets of tuna fish at the theater in case I needed protein during a three-hour rehearsal. Before heading out on an impromptu family trip to see a movie, I'd grab a big chunk of cheese and smear an equally sized gob of peanut butter on it and eat that while walking so I'd have enough protein to get through the movie. No way was the bucket of buttered popcorn and box of Milk Duds going to be able to sustain me through my protein deficiency. A peanut butter cup might supply some protein, but I'd need to eat a few packs of them to get through an epic animated feature.

Fuck you, protein.

For most things that I don't know jack shit about, I have friends who do know precisely jack shit, but not about protein. My friends are just as clueless as the rest of the world. Everyone seems to be drunk on the protein Kool-Aid. There are zillions of "high-protein" diets. There are "low-fat" and "low-carbs," but unless you've got rare genetic kidney cooties, no one is talking about a low-protein diet. When I was learning to cook on TV, every dish had to have its protein. Menus now have protein sections. Everyone is sucking protein's dick.

The way I now understand it (we know this will still be wrong), no food is really protein. Every single goddamn little tiny cell in every single goddamn living organism, plant or animal, has up to 10,000 proteins inside. Every single fucking cell of every single fucking living fucking thing. Proteins really are the building blocks of all life. But that doesn't mean you have to eat a T-bone covered in peanut butter cheese sauce every four hours. In fact, the protein we eat isn't even the protein we use. The protein we use is synthesized by our genes. That's what genes are: recipes for making 25,000 proteins. The DNA in each of our cells makes that shit all the time. We're little peanut butter/ cheese/fish factories. Using amino acids, our cells make all the protein they need.

That's all a protein is: just a sequence of twenty amino acids. (Wikipedia agrees with CrayRay on this—I checked. Some articles say twenty-one amino acids are needed; let's just call it "a bunch.") The order and length of the amino acid sequence gives protein its function and a 3-D shape without clunky 3-D glasses. Everyone makes the comparison to the twenty letters of our alphabet and how those twenty letters make words, sentences, paragraphs, chapters, and books. "Wait just a minute," you say, "we don't have a twenty-letter alphabet, we have a twenty-six-letter alphabet."

And then I say, "Oh, I guess I left out $U R A Q T$!"

And then you say, "That's still only twenty-five."

And I say, "I'll give you the D later."

And then you say, "I guess what you really meant is that there are twenty amino acids, so your analogy to our twenty-six-letter alphabet is off by six, asshole."

We don't use even one single protein from any other organism without first breaking it down into its parts. We eat protein from other animals and plants and break it down into the twenty amino acids, and then use that abbreviated alphabet to build our own protein "words" from the individual "letters." Those amino acids circulate around our bodies in a very small pool of alphabet soup. We don't store amino acids the way we store fat, which is why we need to replenish the supply.

Of those twenty (or so) amino acids, our body synthesizes eleven of them all on its own. Fuck you, protein—we can just make them ourselves. We're like fucking plants—life out of nothing, solar power. We never, ever, ever need to eat any of those eleven, those "nonessential amino acids."

Let's try this analogy. It's as if the alphabet had twenty letters and we could draw eleven of them on our own as long as we had ink and paper, and that ink and paper can come from just about any food. But we couldn't draw the other nine letters, the "essential amino acids," so we had to eat magazines and digest them to break down the words into those nine letters. So we need to find magazines with the nine letters we can't draw. Is that clearer? But those nine letters aren't rare. It's not like we have to find the elusive X, Z, and J—nope, the nine we can't make are like fucking T, H, and E—they're fucking everywhere. You can eat Dickens and Melville, or you can eat the *National Enquirer*, and you'll get plenty of those nine letters that you can use to spell everything your body needs to spell.

The proteins in your body are made of these twenty amino acids, eleven of them in your handwriting, the other nine cut and pasted like a ransom note or an old Sex Pistols album cover. Picture a really stupid kidnapper who cuts out nine letters and then writes all the rest in his own handwriting. No matter how badly read our kidnapper is, he can find those nine letters in whatever hole in the wall he's hiding out in.

We make the eleven nonessential amino acids, so we don't have to worry about them; everyone knows that. But people go bug-nutty over those nine essential amino acids, because we do have to eat those. No animal is able to make all twenty. Every animal needs to eat some amino acids. Only plants make all of them, because plants don't eat (except for Venus flytraps, pitcher plants (we have some in our terrarium with the lizards), Audrey II, and a few others).

To get those nine we eat a plant or we eat an animal that ate a plant, because *only plants make them all*. Every animal we eat to get our essential amino acids got them originally from a plant. Why not go right to the source and ask the horse (I made a bet that I could get a *Mister Ed* reference into this book). Horses don't eat anything but plants, and they build strong bodies that some women find sexy in a way that's a little creepy. The point is that although we do need to eat "protein" to get these nine essential amino acids, we don't need a lot of it, we don't need it often, and we can get it pretty much anywhere. To go back to my old analogy that never really worked, we don't have to swallow the Bible and *Ulysses* every hour to get the letters we need— we can pretty much get them all delivered to our door in a Chick tract that some crazy Christian dropped there. (Chick tracts are those weird little cartoon pamphlet things, printed in black and white in a strange size on really cheap paper, with one color on the cover besides black—usually a washed-out green or orange. They're all about Christ and hell and suffering and dying and feature cartoon people screaming in agony because they didn't have the right kind of faith. If a Chick tract is about evolution, there's always a bug-crazy demonic monkey; that makes me happy. Chick tracts kind of went away with dirty phone booths, but you can still find them once in a while on top of a dirty urinal in a bus station or strip club. Jack Chick, the guy who writes, draws, and prints these little psycho anti-life graphic beat poems, is still alive, and I have it on good authority that he once said, "We need more Christians like Penn Jillette," whatever the holy Jesus with a G-string that fucking means. And I'm very proud he said that, because I'm as fucking crazy as Jack Chick. What I'm trying to explain is that even a small booklet you find on top of a urinal would be likely to have all the letters you need, so you should eat ugly Christian propaganda that you find on top of dirty urinals. I'm here to help.)

We all got into the bad habit of getting our essential amino acids from sources that were a lot like us. Animals concentrate these amino acids in their flesh, so why not eat their asses and get a big dose all at once? That was fine when we were starving and had to get them, along with any calories we could, any way we could manage. Which is to say, it was fine for over a million years. But, as Bob sings, "The times, they are a-changing": we don't need megadoses of these things, and it seems a lot better for us to get them from plants now. Since the beginning of life, for most everybody, the problem was too few calories—but now, for a few of us, the problem is too many calories. Our lizard brains haven't learned that some of us have too many calories. This is a wonderful problem to have. In the United States of America, poor people are too fat! That's amazing. We need to do a little dance and celebrate that. That's hard work, freedom, and technology. YAY! Now let's fix it. We can't eat every meal as though we're not going to eat for another two weeks, and then eat that same mound of fat-fuck food again three hours later. We just can't. And we don't need to concentrate our calories and amino acids. Those essential amino acids that we need to live might also be the very same things that accelerate aging. Fuck! I just slipped that little "accelerate aging" bombshell right up your ass there, didn't I? Yeah, there are a lot of studies that seem to show that massive doses of amino acids age us more rapidly. American medicine has made our deaths much slower, but it hasn't done all that much for extending our healthy lives. It seems to me there's very little we can add to our diet to stay healthier longer, but taking stuff out really seems to help. I'm sixty now; if this shit works, I'll write a book about life extension when I'm eighty-five and still ranting onstage in Vegas.

We have so much food that we don't have to worry much about deficiencies of even the essential amino acids. But we do need to worry about the excess of them. You don't need to think about protein; your body makes it all the time and then pisses it away. Plants have all the amino acids. Our dear friend and lover, the potato, has every single amino acid, and our friend the potato is not special. Rice has all twenty as well. These plants, man, they can make shit. Our bodies are flooded with amino acids all the time. So many more than we need. We try to burn them as fuel, but mostly our organs just work too hard

sorting and sifting and shitting and pissing them away. I don't understand this at all, but it seems that just having too many amino acids on
board can fuck our shit. We're not good at getting rid of them.

So, fuck protein. Eating protein the way all your douche bag
friends want you to will just accelerate your aging and make you a fat
fuck. That's what it did to me.

A TRIP TO THE DOCTOR—
ABOUT HALFWAY THROUGH
COLD AND HUNGRY

I have a good Vegas doctor. That's a rare being. Vegas is good at pole dancers. We import them and we grow them domestically. We have second- and third-generation pole dancers here. We're maggoty with pole dancers. My little girl, Moxie, took dance classes when she was five years old. Her teacher was "Miss Cynthia,"* and she was everything you could want in a little-girl-dance-class teacher. She was skilled, patient, kind, and friendly. Miss Cynthia bubbled. By and by, I got to talking to Miss Cynthia after one of the classes. I asked her how business was, and she said something like, "Good, but I still can't make it just on these classes. I have to keep my night job." She said she danced in one of the local shows. Then it hit me: Miss Cynthia works

---

* "Cynthia" is not her real name. But it's closer to her real name than "Lexi," which is what you called the dancer at Taco Town when you were here last. Oh, and when you met your dancer, it wasn't really her first night, and you didn't really remind her of her brother. She doesn't have a brother, and even if she does, she was still lying to you. Lying is more a part of her job than dancing.

topless! In Vegas, we're all experts on topless. In my zip code, everyone is qualified to do breast exams. There's the fancy "Jubilee" show, which, until it closed in early 2016, was the topless show you'd take your mom to, with costumes that you'd find on special-edition Barbie Dolls; and there's "Taco Town" (I think the real name of the place is Talk of the Town), which you, well, might not take your mom to, unless HBO is doing a late-night documentary on your family. And there's everything in between. Women in Vegas are fully nude from the age of eighteen on, and then when they turn twenty-one, they put thongs on. The reason for that is you can't have pussy and alcohol in the same club. Not unless your naked vagina club is grandfathered in, which is a combination of words that . . . gets a lot of Google Images hits. A young woman dancer in Vegas can make a *lot* more money if there's alcohol around and her breasts are out than if there's no alcohol around. But if there's no alcohol around, then she'd damn well better have everything on display. She can't legally work at a club with alcohol, where she'd just be topless, until she turns twenty-one. So, if you want to see bottomless in Vegas, it's only going to be legal if she's between eighteen and twenty-one. That's creepy to me—and I'm the one who was okay with my daughter taking dance lessons in Vegas. I could tell Miss Cynthia was over twenty-one, and from the way she moved, her height, and her natural dancer body type, I figured Miss Cynthia was at the top of the topless pecking order. I guessed she worked the classy show.

"Yeah, but some of the moms don't like to know that."

"But some of the moms do like to know that, and all of the dads."

So five-year-old Mox was being trained in pole dancing. We turn out great pole dancers in Vegas. Doctors we're not as good at, but after living here for almost two decades, I finally found a good doctor. He works with one of those "concierge" doctor scams. We pay him extra, and he actually gives us appointments. He's a smart guy, and funny and honest and perfectly discreet. You'll never find out from him that I have herpes. He's a pro.

I was over seven weeks into CrayRay's hard-core cold and hungry diet, and I'd dropped about half the weight I had planned to drop. My whole life was changing. I was changing the way I dressed, anticipating the move into something other than XXXL work shirts and big-boy jeans. I wanted to cut my hair and stop dyeing it. I wanted short salt-and-pepper hair. Tom Jones suggested I go with short gray hair. It worked for him, but he's Tom Jones; a pile of dog shit would look good on his head. I'm Penn Jillette; pussy and a Vermeer wouldn't look good on my head.

It was amazing how my life was changing with my eating. Correlation is not causation, and it's more likely the changes were all caused by something I'm not aware of, but with my change in diet came changes in personality, in mood, in desires. Being a Las Vegan was changing everything. EZ and I were even thinking of buying a new house. We wanted to move out of the Slammer, the house that's been featured in a zillion bullshit celebrity stories on me. It was a big, huge nuthouse of bright colors. This house was me, and we were thinking of moving someplace else. Someplace where the children could have friends. When I built the Slammer, I wanted to be isolated from the world. Aside from doing the Penn & Teller show at the Rio, everything I needed or wanted was in my compound. But then I had children, and as a family we didn't want to be isolated. Children want to have friends nearby. But I wasn't open to a new house—not until I was on CrayRay's nutty diet. I woke up happier. I lived happier. I was nicer. Was it just not carrying more extra pounds than my daughter weighed around with me all the time, or was this diet making me happier in other ways? Was it making me more open to change? I don't know.

I showed up at the doctor's office, and the nurse took my weight. She came out with 255, with clothes on, which was lower than my fancy Withings scale said. I'll take it. It might be a part of concierge doctoring services that their scale takes a few pounds off. She took my blood pressure, which was lower than my fancy Withings cuff said, but still not low enough. It was the first time in ten years that she'd taken my blood pressure without wincing, and this was with me no longer taking two of my heavy meds. She smiled. I was proud.

My doctor came in, looked at me, and gave his medical opinion: "Wow."

I said, "Um, this visit isn't really a medical visit. I just came in to brag about my weight loss."

"Yeah, I gathered that when you texted about the appointment. It's not a checkup, and you have no complaints."

"Correct. But I've lost a lot of weight."

"You sure have."

"Neat, huh?"

"Yup. Very neat."

"Okay, good-bye."

I guess that's the way it should have gone, but it went longer. He asked me how I was feeling, and I gave him all the cult stuff. I felt great. I was happier. I had a metric shit-ton of energy. My bowels moved great, my arthritis was better, and my dick got harder and looked bigger. TSA preflight check was going faster. This diet was amazing. All hail CrayRay!

Doc had had other patients lose as much weight as I had in as short a period of time, but they'd always felt terrible. They had no energy and felt really sick. These other thinner people weren't happy and bragging, they were sad and complaining. He said the other fat fucks were doing a "low-carb" diet of some kind. I wasn't doing low carbs. As a matter of fact, CrayRay doesn't even use the word "carbs."

He uses the word "starches." Yes, starches are carbs, but "that's like saying a square is a rectangle." He said that as though it meant that it was stupid to say a square is a rectangle. That's CrayRay's definition of stupid. My definition of stupid is dropping my cock into a hot blow-dryer. My guru is on a higher plane.

I couldn't wait to take my shirt off. I wanted to take my pants off and show my doc how much bigger my cock looked when not nestled in a mound of Crisco. But he didn't need to see my dick. Okay, he wasn't even really willing to see my dick. I tried. He thought my heart sounded great. My lungs sounded great, and I seemed happy. I had no complaints. He had other exam rooms that were full of patients who were really suffering. He seemed to not really have time to celebrate my happy cock. Fuck him.

My blood pressure was still higher than we wanted. I was still jamming at about 170. That's really bad for a normal human, but really good for me or a fat giraffe. And this was with two of my heavy, heavy drugs gone. But I still had to get lower. He told me the system I was using to check my blood pressure at home, which included Mox jumping up and down on my lap while Z blasted video games on his iPad, might not be totally accurate. He said that keeping the cuff on my arm while the children played on me, and testing ten times in a row, was giving me higher readings.

I promised to move my fancy BP cuff from the family room to my office, that I would take my blood pressure just once per sitting, and that I would meditate before I took it. Yup—I was going to meditate.

Meditate?!

Yes, and fuck you in the neck.

While I was still a fat fuck, my buddy Sam Harris had been trying to get me to meditate. I read his book *Waking Up: A Guide to Spirituality Without Religion*. He's such a good writer that I got sucked into

his world. I finished an advance copy of the book in the middle of the
night in the bathtub. I couldn't sleep. My mind was blown. I wrote
to Sam Harris, and to Greg Gutfeld, Richard Dawkins, and Lawrence
Krauss about Sam's book and how it was changing my life. Greg said
my e-mails about Sam's book seemed like they were "haikus written
by a person with Tourette's syndrome." I was gone, daddy, gone. The
idea of the self and the "I," and being in the now and being spiritual
without religion, made me just nuts. I have a very strong sense of
"I." I do feel I'm a homunculus recklessly driving this big old body
from behind my eyes. Sam gave me another way to see things. I was
completely on board the Sam Harris atheist spiritual express bus. I
couldn't sleep.

Dawn came up over the Vegas Strip, and on my phone came
an e-mail from a mutual friend of Bob Dylan's with a link to Dylan
doing a version of a Sinatra song. I listened to "Full Moon and
Empty Arms" done in a different kind of world-weary voice from
Frank's and a five-piece band playing the orchestra arrangement in
the cold bathtub with no sleep to soothe my brain, and . . . well,
if Bob Dylan was recording songs made famous by Frank Sinatra,
then maybe Penn, or this living thing in this exact moment, could
be spiritual. Maybe Sam Harris had written a BB gun of a book that
could shoot my "I" out.

As dawn turned to morning and spiritual Vegas became the fucking desert, I got e-mails back from Lawrence and Dawkins, and over
the next few weeks some of Sam's mind bending fell away. But Sam
is such a good writer that while I was reading his book, and for a few
weeks afterward, I was completely on the spiritual bandwagon. But
as I got further away from having taken in the words on my iPad, it
seemed that the experiences he refers to as "spiritual" became more
and more like Sam just loved LSD. That's certainly valid, but I'm not
sure it's really spiritual. It also seems that his form of meditation is

believe Muhammad was any sort of prophet. I don't believe there are any real prophets. That idea is wrong. And if I say that idea is wrong, that doesn't mean I have an irrational fear of people who believe that idea. It means that I think the idea is wrong, wrong, wrong. And I'm a bit scared of spiders.

Sam is a hippie peacenik who's not preaching hate, he's preaching dropping acid and not talking to people in India. So, I decided to give meditation another try, in order to get my blood pressure down and get back to the business of losing weight so my dick would look bigger.

Sam writes about all the wondrous upsides of meditation. He talks a lot about relieving stress. I don't feel I have much stress. I'm not a worrier, but I have high blood pressure, so maybe I'm a secret worrier. Maybe I worry without knowing it. Maybe there's some low-blood-pressure bliss that I'm missing.

Sam sent me a recording of him talking me through a guided mindfulness meditation. I was trying to do it every day before the show. I would go into my dressing room and get caught up on all my e-mail and then close the door, put on headphones, and do what Sam told me to do. Again, I was doing that when I was a fat fuck, and I kind of liked it okay, but it didn't do that much for me. Then I got busy again, and getting my self to fall away fell away. But now I was down fifty pounds and off some of the BP medicine, and I was happier and stronger and . . . what the hell, it's supposed to help blood pressure, so I could give Sam ten minutes and get myself on the bus to Nirvana, and then slip on the BP cuff and see how I did.

I love things like blood pressure measurement, because there are no subjective rules. You're allowed to cheat all you want. There's no judgment call. You can do anything you want to get it as low as you want. One of the many things I hate about magic is all the judgment calls. Yeah, you can certainly be smoother as a juggler and make the built to fix problems I don't have. He writes a lot about needing to get rid of the voice that's in his head, the sense of self that makes him crazy. I like the voices in my head. My sense of self gives me a sense of self. I like it. By going to India and not talking for months (why talk in India? Those fucks can't understand you anyway) and dropping acid, he lost the sense of self that had been making him nuts. His book is about how to do that. It's fun to read, and it made me wonderfully crazy in the bathtub in the middle of the night, but maybe I don't want to do that. If you're reading this book and you're not overweight at all, you don't have to join a cult and lose weight. As a matter of fact, if you're fucking obese, you don't have to join a cult and lose weight. You bought my book, and that's it—you don't owe me jack shit. Go to India and drop acid, for all I care.

Sam Harris is just a hippie. He's as hippie as they come. He's more of a hippie than me, and that's saying something. And Sam the hippie gets accused by Ben Affleck of being "Islamaphobic." Oh, the joy I felt at my spell checker not recognizing "Affleck" or "Islamaphobic"! (Just for the record, my spell checker recognizes both "Elvis" and "Arachnophobia." You know why that is? Because Elvis is really a superstar, and spiders are really fucking scary.) Being "Muslimphobic" would be a really bad thing. That would be like being "homophobic" (also in my spell checker, but not a very pleasant word; it always seems like it means "fear of same," and that's just not what it is). "Homophobic" has come to mean fear of people who are gay. That would be like "Muslimphobic" meaning a fear of a kind of person, and that would be awful. But Islam is not a kind of person. Islam is an idea. Islam is a religion. And religions are not people. Ideas are not people. All ideas must be attacked all the time, in order to find out what parts of them are true. We must respect people, but that doesn't mean we have to respect ideas that aren't true. I don't even care whether the ideas are dangerous or not. I don't care if Islam does mean "peace." I don't tricks look better, but if you're not bent over looking like you're chasing a duck while you pick up the props you dropped—if the balls are in the air—you're kind of doing the trick okay. When you're learning magic, there are all these judgment calls. I'm learning this new false shuffle called the Truffle Shuffle. It looks like the deck is being shuffled normally, but all the cards stay in the same order in the deck. It's a shuffle that does no shuffling. That's a useful technique in magic. Now, the first few steps of learning this shuffle are just juggling: I have to do the move without the cards falling on the floor or changing order. I can check that. I can work on that. The hard step is the next step, the most important step: to "make it look natural." When I was juggling, impossibly passing nine clubs with Mike Moschen when I was twenty, we did not want to look natural—we wanted to look as unnatural as fucking a male rhino in a skirt. That's the point of learning an amazing juggling trick. But in magic, the hardest moves are supposed to look natural, so you work for years to look like you're doing nothing. That's way unnatural.

Taking your blood pressure is juggling. You can do any cheat you want to get it as low as possible, and that's your reading. So maybe I didn't have to diet at all; maybe I could stay fat and just drop acid in India with Sam Harris and bring my BP down to a healthy level.

Every night I'd been taking a bunch of analgesics for the arthritis in my thumbs. The hardest physical part of the show for me is when I display the .357 Magnum bullet between my index finger and thumb. That just kills me. I try to tell people that the arthritis came from how much I practiced juggling and sleight of hand, but that's not true. And then I lie to myself and figure it's genetic, but that's never true. When I take analgesics, I take a lot. I figure I'm twice the size of a normal person, so I need twice the dose, and then I figure doses are low on the label, so maybe three times will do. My doc told me,

"Don't take Advil, it's bad for your blood pressure," but then he told me I was in BP denial, so when the aspirin ran out I moved to Advil and was taking four times the dose and doing it every night to get my thumbs to hold a fucking bullet to shoot my business partner in the face. Then I started losing weight like a freak and my thumbs didn't hurt as much, but I was still taking the Advil out of habit. All of a sudden I cared about my health, so I asked the doc if there was any way the Advil could be bringing up my blood pressure.

"Well, you stupid fucking fat fuck, it could be that it is, since I told you it would and it says it will on the fucking label and you're overdosing on it like a fucking asshole," is not what my doctor said. He said, "Yes, by maybe twenty points. Stop taking the Advil."

So I stopped the overdose of Advil and went to an underdose of aspirin. Amazingly, with the weight loss, I hardly needed it for my thumbs. I ate a metric shit-ton of greens and took my blood pressure in my quiet office after meditating instead of while children were jumping on me. My idea of meditation is listening to the calming ding of my computer getting messages and thinking about what I'm going to write in this book when I'm supposed to be thinking about breathing, and still my blood pressure, with no Advil, more greens, and a little quiet, was . . . 134/74. So there.

I've tried a few more ways to meditate. I liked Sam's recording, but I started to memorize it. Then this company called Headspace .com started advertising on *Penn's Sunday School*, so I was being paid to be mindful. I found that if I didn't think the word "meditate" but changed it to "be mindful," I didn't feel as silly. Now I'm doing ten minutes a day of Headspace.com, and I can't memorize it because it changes every day, and it has goals, and I feel like I'm starting to get it. Sam told me I would have to start and stop a few times before it caught. I'm back to doing it again, and it feels like it's sticking. My BP is down, but I'm not sure that's the mindfulness, because my body continues to heal and get better from my diet, but it might be giving me more control. I don't know. But it's nice to sit and play with my head a bit.

Sam and Headspace.com are interesting and fun . . . but I think the BP fix is all CrayRay.

FROM HALFWAY TO ALL THE WAY

DAY 48: 256.7

I suppose the food I was eating, and still eat, qualifies as "bland." But very spicy. Maybe "bland" just means not much salt, sugar, and fat. The diet had changed my senses, and what qualifies as "bland" was surprisingly flavorful. I could taste vegetables. Celery tasted salty! My sense of smell was better, and now I cared about smells. I liked the subtle healthy smells of food being cooked. I started burning scented candles in my office while I worked. I was becoming a fucking hippie.

Every night, after every Penn & Teller show we've ever done, Teller and I go out and meet the audience. If anyone wants something signed, we sign it. It's become popular lately for other shows to charge an extra hundred bucks for a "VIP Meet and Greet," and the entertainers will meet only with anyone who's paid the extra jingle. Well, everyone is a VIP with us. We don't do it to offer "added value," we do it because we like it. It seems that if people like our show, it's likely we'll like them. Doing this for forty years has made us different from other entertainers. The only feedback other performers get is onstage, so if a crowd is quiet, other entertainers are bummed. But we go out and talk to people, and often the quietest crowds contain the people who are the most enthusiastic and kind when we meet them after the show, when it's one on one. When I'm seeing a show, the better it is, the quieter I am. I can barely bring myself to applaud when I'm watching Dylan. I'm afraid to lose my concentration, to break the spell. After forty years, Teller and I have grown to trust and enjoy the quiet audiences. You could point out that this is a self-selected sample—that the people who come up to us and wait to meet us are the few people who liked the show, while the rest of the quiet crowd really hated us. You could say that, and you might be right, but you'd be a prick.

So everyone gets VIP treatment at our show. Some entertainers thought we did this for business reasons and that it explained the success we've had, so they tried it, but they stopped after a while. It doesn't seem that you can do this if you don't love it and really love your audience. On our last run on Broadway, meeting everyone after the show got to be too hectic and crazy, and a couple of times the post-show lasted longer than the show-show, so we had to make it more organized. We were out there for over ninety minutes. When we played the Hammersmith Apollo in London, every night we were meeting people for longer than we'd been onstage. The theater staff would close up and go home, and we'd be out on the street with our audience in the dark, except for cell phone camera flashes. We loved it. Some entertainers will sign only their own merchandise. We'll sign anything. We've signed more than a couple arms and backs for our signatures to be turned into tattoos. I always feel guilty at how shitty my writing is when that happens. Since there are two of us, and breasts often come in pairs, we've signed a bunch of those, and Teller draws a nice ampersand on the lady's chest between the tit flesh. I've only signed a couple of cocks, but I still think about ways to make it say "Penn & Teller" when flaccid and then "Penn is the tall one who talks & Teller is the shorter one who doesn't really talk all that much" when aroused. If more men asked us, we'd work that out.

If anyone in the crowd wants to take a picture with us, we pose with them. Teller billboards himself to people as "the King of Selfies," and he takes pictures for them like a politician. I like to encourage cooperation among strangers, so I have people hand their cameras to a stranger to take the picture. We pretend that people can talk to us during this process, but the awareness that other people are waiting cuts off conversation, unless people hang out for over an hour until everyone is gone—but the crew is waiting backstage to get my mics and suit off so they can go home, so chat time is kind of limited to "You were better than I thought you were going to be."

My diet changed the post-show. All of a sudden I could really smell people. I could smell their perfume, hair-care products, soaps, and breath. I never noticed that stuff before the diet, but now I was really aware of it, and it bothered me. It distracted me. There isn't that much to be distracted from; I'm just saying "Thanks, boss" over and over again while looking at people. I hope no one ever catches me, but my thoughts are not chaste while I look at attractive people in our audience. If you come to see our show and you come up to me afterward to get something signed or to take a picture, you can bet your well-imagined ass that at the very least, I'm picturing you naked. Since there's usually no formal queue but just people gathered around, I have some control over who comes up next for his or her picture. If I find you really attractive, I'll skip over you a few times so I can keep looking at you while posing with other people. You get punished if I find you attractive. That's the kind of guy I am.

I've always been worried about how I smell after the show, so I'd invariably suck on a Ricola lozenge, figuring it was better to smell like cough drops than a ninety-minute monologue with a fire-eating gasoline finish. CrayRay put an end to the Ricola. It's just sugar that I don't need. So I discovered breath strips, those little brightly colored Listerine pieces of weird-ass plastic that dissolve in your mouth. I found that if I stuck five of them in my mouth as I was running through the crowd, the flavor of them would overwhelm my sense of smell, and I wouldn't be bugged by audience members smelling like people.

Once I discovered breath strips, I also discovered breath sprays, and I got to love those, too. A burst of flavor without eating anything. These turned into my snacks. I was eating once a day, but I'd have decaffeinated coffee, tea, breath strips, and spray anytime—yum, a banquet.

DAY 51: 254.1

DAY 53: 255.6

I was plateauing at a high weight for me. I went back up a few pounds and stayed there for a couple of days. After all this progress it was discouraging, but even at this "high" weight, I was still lower than I could remember being. Years ago I appeared on *Dancing with the Stars*. We weren't allowed to take dancing lessons before going on (I believe I was the only one who followed that rule), but we were allowed to exercise and diet. Using a grown-up stupid diet consisting of a lot of protein, calorie counting, and a ton of exercise, I got myself down below 260 for a minute and was in pretty good shape. It was really hard to get down there, and I went right back up after I lost, and I lost quickly—I was the first one off the show. It was the best shape I'd been in for years, and I felt great (although I was still on all my blood pressure meds then; it wasn't the right kind of weight loss to help that). I really thought 260 would be my lowest weight, and now, riding with CrayRay, it seemed like 229 wasn't out of the question. Mind blowing.

DAY 54: 251.3

A very nice correction. I was down where I expected to be, and right back on track. My Withings software tracked my weight and told me what I would have to do per day to hit my goal. I'd set my goal to weigh 229 pounds by my sixtieth birthday, March 5, 2015. That would be down to the lowest weight I could find in my diaries, back in the '80s Off-Broadway.

DAY 55: 252.2

They say the two happiest days in a man's life are the day he buys his boat and the day he sells his boat. For me, one of the happiest days was the day I got my CPAP machine, and I was looking forward to the day I could get rid of it. The CPAP is a fat-guy machine. The CPAP machine delivers Continuous Positive Airway Pressure while you're sleeping. Before I got the CPAP, I went for years without getting one good night's sleep. I never really got too much REM. I was exhausted and depressed all the time. My doc finally sent me to a sleep clinic. The woman at the clinic who was sticking all sorts of pads, gizmos, and wires all over my face, head, and chest looked different from the woman I had hoped would be watching me sleep. There were scheduling problems because I don't go to sleep until after 3:00 a.m. and it fucked up everyone's shifts, but I have my picture on the side of a building, so I got special treatment. Still, my picture on the side of a building wasn't big enough for me to get the woman I had hoped for to put me to sleep. My sleep doctor was pretty freaked by how many times I woke up each hour. My nights were not spent knitting up the ravell'd sleeve of care but rather choking on my own fat. He prescribed a CPAP. He said he loved prescribing CPAPs, because people really did get better overnight.

And I did get better overnight. The CPAP stopped my apnea. It stopped my fat neck from cutting off my air while I slept and choking me awake every minute or so. The CPAP kept constant air pressure so I could breathe all night and finally sleep. They did another sleep study (this time a small Asian man put me to sleep; closer to my fantasy, but still not dead-on) and I was in REM the whole night. I was singing with an Athens, Georgia, band. It was the best I'd ever felt before going on the diet. I loved, loved, loved my CPAP. It didn't make me attractive in bed, but it sure gave me my dreams back. I bought a bunch of them and had them sent to the hotels where I would be staying so I wouldn't have to take them through TSA checks. I kept one permanently at my favorite hotel in L.A.

I loved my CPAP. I would strap it on when it was time to sleep and it would start its gentle breeze, and off I would drift. I loved the sound and the feeling and even the straps around my head. They were a trigger for comfort and sleep. But as I lost weight, the CPAP changed. What used to feel like a gentle summer breeze as I slept was now blowing the nose off my face. I was choking in the other direction. It felt like I was trying to breathe in a hurricane. Then they came out with a new machine that automatically adjusts to the air pressure you need. EZ sleeps next to me, and she's heard the machine go from hurricane down to very gentle breeze.

As of this writing I've been at my target weight for six months, and I'm still using the CPAP. It's barely on, but I still love it and want it. The docs all say that in the next year the CPAP will go away, along with the rest of the meds. I'm looking forward to sleeping like a thin guy. The two happiest days in a fat fuck's life: the day he gets his CPAP and the day he gets rid of his CPAP.

DAY 57: 250.6

I had to fly to NYC. There was no airplane food that was going to be acceptable, so I went to a Chinese restaurant at the airport where they had plain rice. I got two orders of that and then went to the Mexican restaurant at the food court and copped a bunch of hot sauce. I hate the plastic bag carry-on, but I took that on the plane, and when it was suppertime, I pulled it out and had cold rice for supper. According to *Apocalypse Now*, all I needed to add was some rat meat and I could be Charlie. The horror, the horror.

I got in and met with Lawrence O'Donnell. We usually go to a restaurant and talk politics. This time we went to his room and talked diet.

The next day I went out with friends. We went to a wonderful fancy Mediterranean restaurant. It was food that I would have considered healthy just months ago—lots of fish and olive oil and bread. But now it seemed like just pools of salt and fat. I had steamed vegetables, and for a real treat I had some beets. At first I was missing my taramasalata. Taramasalata (I'm putting that word in the book twice in a row so I can read it twice in a row for the audiobook. My buddy Christian Bök wrote a book called *Eunoia*, and each chapter is univocalic—another word I look forward to reading aloud—meaning each chapter uses only one vowel. It has sentences like "A law as harsh as a fatwa bans all paragraphs that lack an *A* as a standard hallmark." And taramasalata is featured in this great sentence: "Hassan wants Kalamata shawarma, cassabananas, and taramasalata." If you think that's great, check out his *U* chapter—you can whack to that one) . . .

anyway, taramasalata is salted fish eggs in creamy gunk. I loved it, but I loved it because it was just salt and fat. Because it's yucky fish eggs, no one else ordered it, so I wasn't tempted. All the food looked wonderful and fresh, but once the conversation started I was happy with my vegetables.

I had to catch a plane to fly home for the Father/Daughter Valentine's Day dance. I got to Vegas in time to pick up Mox at school. The VD dance had an '80s theme this year, so EZ crimped Mox's hair, and she looked all Cyndi Lauper. I put on some of the clothes I wore in the Run-DMC video we shot back in the '80s that now fit me again, and off we went to the dance with all the other fathers and daughters. We got our picture taken and I bought her flowers, all the up-sells the school does to make more money. Who cares? We danced together, and although it wasn't '80s, we sang "All About that Bass" together. Mox is small for nine years old, so we can still slow dance with me holding her off the floor, and we jumped around together, and at my new weight, I could really jump around. I'm not saying I could keep up with nine-year-olds, but I sure could go longer than my 330-pound fat-fuck self. We were there for the whole event, and she stepped up to the mic and said, "I love you, Daddy," as part of that tradition. Yeah, I cried—you got a problem with that?

We went home, and Mox asked if we could go outside and look at the stars. We laid on the couch in the courtyard and looked up together. We talked about time and distance and how long the light took to reach us, and then we talked about my mom and dad and sister and how hard they worked and what they meant to me and how much I missed them. I talked about traits Mox has that are like those my dad and my mom had. It was a time to be treasured. And as we spoke of my mom, dad, and sister, it was hard not to think that they all died of illnesses related to diet. Maybe I'll be around a little longer for my little girl because I didn't eat the taramasalata (and now I get to say it again on the audiobook). Mox was tired, and I took off my coat and she laid on my chest and I put the coat over both of us. She fell asleep on my chest, and I slept a little, too, but I also just enjoyed it. After about an hour I carried her upstairs and put her to bed. She weighs just about half the amount of weight I'd lost, so carrying her up the stairs was about the same as just walking my own fat-fuck ass up the stairs less than three months before. Goddamn.

DAY 63: 247.2

DAY 64: 248.6

DAY 65: 246.5

I have 17.5 pounds to go in twenty-four days. It's going to be close.

DAY 66: 246.3

DAY 67: 247.8

The children wanted to go outside and play, and I just jumped up and did it. I did it when I was a fat fuck, too, but it took a lot of saying to myself, "Time goes so fast; this is a chance to play with your children, and you don't want to miss it." But it was so easy at this weight. We played tetherball and I was really into it. I pushed Z on the scooter and fell down on top of him, but I was light enough now that holding my weight above my son without crushing him was easy. We all laughed about our "epic fail"; six months ago, it would have meant a trip to the hospital. It's great to not be so fat that moving isn't fun. I was really able to play with my children. Kind of a big deal.

DAY 68: 246.9

DAY 69: 245.6

DAY 71: 244.6

CrayRay had warned Goudeau and me that we'd hit a point where people would say how great and healthy we looked, and shortly afterward would start telling us we'd lost enough and we were now looking gaunt and unhealthy. It began with one of my L.A. buddies, who said, "Okay, now cool it, you're starting to look sick; you've done it, now go back to eating normal." CrayRay had predicted it. He says in some cases, friends and family try interventions and get doctors on board to tell the person to start eating. They throw around words they don't understand, like "anorexia." Anorexia (I'm repeating that, but not for the audiobook; it's not a fun word to say) is a serious medical condition and is not tied in with our weight loss. We might be stupid, but we're not sick.

We did the *Penn's Sunday School* podcast. We had read about snorting chocolate and talked about it on the show, and someone in Canada, where it's being sold, sent us some. It had fancy packaging and a little spring-loaded double nasal catapult. Goudeau cocked it and put two little coke-spoons full of their fancy chocolate-and-spice mixture in it, one on each side, and I held it under my nose, breathed in, and hit the button. We had checked with CrayRay, and he said it wouldn't affect the diet, but it probably wasn't healthy. I love chocolate, and I got a big blast of it up my nose and down into my lungs. I kinda wanted to love it. The idea that I'd be snorting chocolate in my office while I was writing this appealed to me. It was a little fun, but really no more fun than walking into a Godiva store at a mall. It was the good smell of chocolate, and that was about it. We all tried it and enjoyed it a little, and then the headaches hit and we were done. I got to the show that night and was light-headed from not eating, and my throat and voice were fucked-up from snorting chocolate. I'm an idiot.

Matt Donnelly, who does the *Penn's Sunday School* podcast with Goudeau and me, sure noticed our weight loss. He has two babies, he's much younger than us, and he's been a fat fuck his whole life. As young as he was, he was already on lots of blood pressure meds and was really worried about how long he was going to be around for his children. Goudeau and I weren't allowed to talk about our weight loss, but Matt was begging us. CrayRay isn't a diet guru, but he's the man with the plan. I called him up and asked him to help our buddy Matt.

I took Matt to the Apple Store and bought him a couple of presents for his newborns. I bought him a Withings scale and blood pressure cuff. If he was going to do it, he was going to do it right. Ray started working with him.

DAY 72: 242.9

We still weren't supposed to exercise, but we felt so fucking good that we had to move. I've always done everything I could to get out of exercising, but now I was running to my car and taking stairs two at a time. When the children suggested any activity, I would jump up to join them. Sixty pounds is a lot of weight not to carry. Goudeau and I wanted to try riding our trikes again. CrayRay said we were allowed to be active, that we could take a nice trike ride, but we shouldn't push it. No real "exercise." We got all Don Johnson, assholes who thought we were groovy, and rode around Goudeau's neighborhood. We weren't supermen. We'd gotten a lot lighter, but also a bit weaker. The balance was still in our favor, but it wasn't magic. We had a nice ride and a talk. Before, when we used to ride, I used to push myself, thinking that if I just rode a little harder for an hour, I would get thinner and feel a little less like I was about to die every second of my life. That compulsion was gone. Now I was just enjoying being outdoors in the desert, chatting with a buddy and loving being alive in my new body. Hey, that ain't bad.

EZ and I were still looking for a new home that would be better for the children. One house that we looked at had fruit and nut trees. I texted CrayRay and got his advice on trying one of the lemons and one of the black walnuts. He said that wouldn't set me back at all, so I did that. Just a couple of mouthfuls, but it was wonderful.

It may seem silly that I was checking with CrayRay over a mere mouthful, but it really matters. I have a great buddy and coworker in NYC. He was a sick fat fuck and wanted to lose weight. He started following Dr. Joel Fuhrman's *End of Dieting* diet and lost some weight and felt better. (Fuhrman is better known in my house as Fuhrburger, and by the time you finish this book, that's how you'll think of him, too.) Then he started thinking, "Well, a little cream in my coffee isn't going to really fuck me up." And then: "Well, I can have a couple of shrimp on my salad at the club." Pretty soon he was shocked and depressed to discover that he wasn't losing weight and wasn't feeling as well. We're not talking homeopathy bullshit here. The memory dilution of a bacon bit is not going to end your life, but it doesn't take much to fuck up the cootie balance in your guts. And it doesn't take much to feel like a grade school child being punished instead of like a nut being hard-core. Mouthfuls matter.

It's essential that I feel like a nut and not a weasel. I must. A nut calls someone to get permission to put one kernel of nut in his mouth. A weasel has a little soy milk in his coffee. The difference is everything to me. Everyone else wanted me to diet like a weasel, with "cheat days" and treats and things I "deserved" that wouldn't make any difference. A nut is hard-core. A nut is beautiful. Bob Dylan is a nut; Hillary Clinton is a weasel. Maybe you want to be Hillary—she changed the world and got a lot of power; but I want to be Bob, so I'll do this fucking right.

DAY 73: 241.4

DAY 74: 241.1

DAY 75: 241.9

I started trying to add three pounds of steamed spinach with my "with the mother"-fucking vinegar to my supper before the show. CrayRay pointed out that spinach is kind of junk food. Yup—I'd gotten to the point where I was too healthy for spinach. He wanted me to try mustard greens and kale. Mustard greens are amazing. Green vegetables with built-in horseradish kick. I loved them. Spinach was still easier to get, and although not bursting with as many nutrients, it certainly wasn't a Big Mac. With the spinach in my stomach, I tried eating a little less of the corn/bean stew and rice.

I felt great, but I was still light-headed during the show. Throughout the *Penn & Teller Show* we use a couple dozen audience members. Some of them are just onstage to hold hands around Elsie while we make that African Spotted Pygmy Elephant vanish, and some are onstage with just Teller, but with most of the rest of them, I ask their names, learn them, and use their names throughout the show. With my light-headedness, I was forgetting their names. My mind would be racing, and I'd hear their names, but when it was time to repeat them, I'd have a zillion more things on my mind and would have to ask them for their names again. That had happened before, but it was rare. Now, on my diet, it was common. I was asking people to repeat their names a lot.

My lack of calories wasn't making me sluggish and stupid. It wasn't giving me headaches or a gnawing grumbling in my stomach. That's what happens on other diets. This CrayRay thing had me speeding. If you want a just-so story from evolution, well, the animals that lack calories and just lie down all crabby and depressed are going to starve right where they are. The animals that lack calories and bubble with energy and new ideas and feel like running around are more likely to find the calories they need and to live longer, fuck more, and pass those hungry-dancing genes on to the next generation. The problem during the show was that I was feeling too good; my mind was racing. I had too many ideas to keep all the stuff I needed to do my job in my head. That's right—I'm trying to pass off being scatterbrained as a survival skill.

I had crossed a line. Teller wrote me an e-mail pointing out that I was missing audience members' names in the show and "going up" on my lines now and again. This was a very heavy e-mail. Teller and I have been partners for forty years, and we don't bust each other on anything. When we're working on a bit we argue about everything and talk about how everything sucks, but once a bit is up on its feet and it's in the show, we trust each other to do our best job. We know that we're both working on making the show better. To send an e-mail saying, essentially, "You're fucking up" is nuclear. I want to stress that his e-mail could not have been more measured and polite; Teller is the perfect business partner and artist, but the very existence of the e-mail was a baseball bat to my face.

I was losing weight and feeling wonderful, but I was fucking up our show. I was losing my focus. I wrote back to Teller and said that I knew I was fucking up, and it was the diet, and I wanted to get through it but I would try to focus better and I was sorry.

He wrote back what he was supposed to write back, that no apology was necessary, he was just worried about me. Damn; at least he could have had the common courtesy to be an asshole about it. I went into the show that night prepared to be perfectly focused. I was going to show that I was just as good as ever. I was going to be articulate and focused and remember all the names and not fuck up. I got through the first three lines of the show—"Good evening, my name is Penn Jillette, and this is my partner, Teller; we are Penn & Teller"—and then stumbled and lost my place and mangled the words. I got our first new friend onstage and forgot her name right away. I'd psyched myself right out. It was still a good show. I don't think the audience thought I was fucking up, but Teller knew, and that meant I really needed to pull it together. I had to get more potatoes or glucose or something on board. I was off a couple more blood pressure drugs—I was doing great—but I couldn't fuck up the show and fuck Teller and our audiences. Fuck.

DAY 77: 237.7

We started planning my birthday party twelve days out. I was originally going to have a big blowout with hamburgers, bacon, doughnuts, hot fudge, ice cream, and fried chicken—just really go nuts. Eat myself sick. That's what had seemed right when I began, but now it didn't seem like what I wanted at all. Now I wanted to get all my friends together and have a meal that would feature all the wonderful food I would eat for the rest of my life. I wanted there to be no animal products, no refined grains, and stupid-low levels of salt, sugar, and oil. We thought about doing it in L.A. because I would be shooting *Sharknado 3* there and I have a lot of friends in L.A. EZ called Jet Tila to find the perfect chef, and started sniffing around for a place to have it.

DAY 78: 237.9

DAY 79: 234.8

DAY 80: 234.7

DAY 81: 234.3

DAY 82: 233.3

It was the final week, and that was a very good weight. So close. I wanted to try to come in lower, but that's really good. I decided to do a couple of days of just greens, so I could make my goal a little early. It would be nice to hit 229 and just be done with it.

I was so close to my target weight, and my birthday was so close that I did something I never do. I went clothes shopping. EZ, the long-suffering Glenn, and I went to a really fancy, expensive shop, and I bought pants. Remember, I started out with size 44 pants, and even on a good day they were too tight. Now a 36 was loose enough to tuck in a shirt without undoing the pants, and I wanted to tuck in my shirts. I tried to find a black silk polka-dotted shirt like Dylan wore in *Don't Look Back*. I'm not young enough or thin enough or hip enough, but I am fuck-you enough. We couldn't find it anyway. I can't remember ever enjoying shopping for clothes, but I did that day. I used to think clothes didn't fit me because I was six foot seven, but that was only part of it. Maybe the bigger part was the fat-fuck part, and I had that pretty much licked.

DAY 84: 229.8

Bingo!

That's it!

I made it!

With five days to spare. This is what it looks like:

On October 10, 2014, I weighed 320.6 pounds. I lost 16.3 pounds on my own, being a grown-up, in fifty-nine days. That's .27 pounds a day, and that's not bad. On December 8, 2014, I weighed 304.3 pounds, and I became a CroNut. On February 28, 2015, I weighed 229.8 pounds. The 320-pound starting weight was not my heaviest. At my heaviest I was over 330, but I didn't weigh myself much then; why would I? But with a combo of being a grown-up and Ray, I'd lost 90.8 pounds in 141 days. That's .64 pounds a day, and that's not just okay, that's amazing. I'd lost 28 percent of my body weight.

But this book is mostly about how I did it with CrayRay, and that's where the numbers get really good. The fattest of the fat is the easiest to get off, and I did that by myself. The CrayRay figures look like this: On December 8, I weighed 304.3 pounds, and on February 28, I weighed 229.8 pounds. In eighty-two days I'd lost 74.5 pounds. That's 0.9 pounds a motherfuckingcuntlapping day!

I had lost 24.5 percent of my body weight in eighty-three days.

Now to start the hard part.

RARE AND APPROPRIATE—
MY TRICK FOR DIETING
WITHOUT TRICKS

I very much enjoy stating that I have never had a drink of alcohol or a toke of any recreational drug in my life. What I don't state is that I will never have a drink of alcohol or a toke of any recreational drug in my life. I can report on the past, but I'm reluctant to predict the future. The hippies were right about fresh vegetables and staying away from fast food, so maybe they're right about LSD. What the fuck do I know? I don't even trust myself completely on the past. I remember things wrong all the time. I'm not willing to say I'm never going to do recreational heroin, so I'm sure as shooting not going to close the Big Mac door forever. I'd like to say that I'll never be a fat fuck again, but I'm not sure of that. I try to take promises, even to myself, seriously. I've got the Fuhrman diet under control. EZ cooks me great food, and I don't even have many cravings for shitty food anymore, but I'm not going to say that any food is off my table for good.

CrayRay conducts experiments himself and keeps up with all the other scientists. But none of this stuff I'm about to write about has really been proven yet. Diet is complicated, and it'll be a long time before we know enough for certain. Ray ran an experiment on himself in which he ate all he could once a week during suppertime, say from 8:00 p.m. to midnight every Friday. Something like that. He sometimes hit six thousand calories in one four-hour window. A couple of times he ate until he puked, and then ate some more. He did stupid gluttony every Friday evening until midnight, and then went right back on hard-core Fuhrburger for the rest of the week. He did this for a good long while and didn't gain any weight. He didn't experience any other ill health effects, either, but this is CrayRay just monkeying around. This wasn't in a lab, so we don't know what he was fucking up that he couldn't or didn't measure. Ray would never report this publicly until he has real, replicable experiments. He's a scientist; he wants real data and real information. But he talks to his buddy Penn, who is not a scientist. Vegas dipshit Penn will report anything to anyone, no matter how half-assed. Ray isn't saying anything on the subject of bingeing yet; this is all Penn. You are getting this health information from a juggler. When CrayRay did this to himself, he ate wholesome foods on these fatty Fridays—he wasn't slamming Big Macs and doughnuts. He was doing high-calorie, but not SAD. So an unreliable juggler is reporting to you that one guy—a really smart guy, but still just one guy—ate a wicked lot once a week and didn't get fatter.

Then CrayRay did another nonreplicable experiment that he himself would never report, but I don't give a fuck, so I will: he added a "treat" every day. He ate perfectly all day, all week, except for a few hundred calories' worth of treat once a day. He'd have a couple of Oreos or something like that. Now, when CrayRay had this small treat every day, his weight started sneaking up. He was gaining weight. Soon CrayRay will do these experiments properly—he'll report his findings in peer-reviewed journals and people will really know this stuff—but as of this writing, it's just me speculating. It's not a scientist's speculation but a Las Vegas magician's speculation on science he knows nothing about. Based on this information, I am sure I can have a shit-ton of bacon and doughnuts every two weeks.

I've taken CrayRay's little experiment and extrapolated it to nonsense. Ray came up with the phrase "Rare and Appropriate" for this idea, and I love it. My thinking—and I repeat, this is based on nothing that's really scientific—is that the body is really good at handling bingeing and not good at all at handling things that are chronic, and what follows is my personal take on "Rare and Appropriate."

In his experiment, CrayRay was eating like a pig once a week. Fuhrburger, in an early book, writes (please remember, I'm paraphrasing, distorting, and misremembering) that your health will stay fine if you get 10 percent of your calories from shit. I decided for myself that I would have Rare and Appropriate no more often than once every two weeks. Two weeks is double the interval CrayRay tried, and I'd be eating even less shit than Fuhrburger's allowable 10 percent. I would wait a minimum of two weeks, and then I would eat whatever I wanted.

I'm writing all around the barn here to avoid saying that every two weeks I'm going to have a cheat day. Motherfucker, I hate that phrase: "cheat day." I really hate it. CrayRay *REALLY* hates it. It's not cheating. My rules include eating like a sick pig every couple of weeks, so I'm not cheating, I'm playing by my rule. I have an open marriage with my diet. We have an understanding. We have an arrangement. My diet is fine with me banging the shit out of pulled-pork tacos now and again. My diet knows it doesn't mean anything. Every two weeks I'm a culinary Russell Brand, and then I go back to being . . . um . . . someone who is known for not fucking, which is . . . um . . . no one. But I'm him or her, whoever that is.

I have a note file on my computer called R&A, and in there I write down when I last ate like a sick pig, so I always know when I'm past my two weeks and have an R&A available. I came up with this plan while I was still in my loss phase. The plan was really important to me. I'd see all my brothers and sisters on MovieNight eating bacon and brownies and I'd think to myself, "Once I hit my target weight, every two weeks I'll eat all of this and more." It made things easier, thinking "not never, just not now." And when I finally reached my target weight, I thought about what my R&A would be. When Penn & Teller were booked on Broadway, I knew I'd have corned beef, pastrami, cheesecake, egg creams, Cel-Ray, Ray's pizza (man, there's a lot of "Rays" in food, huh?), bagels, cream cheese, lox, and soft serve. I'd be able to have all of that during a six-week run, but I wouldn't have it every day or even every week. I could easily go to NYC and not eat any of that, but it would be hard to know I was going to go to NYC and not eat any of that at all. It's pretty easy to not eat something right now when I know I'll be eating it in the future.

I hit my target weight by my sixtieth birthday, March 5, 2015. That was the day I went from losing to maintenance—but it was also my birthday, so not only did I have the stuff I would soon be eating every day for the first time in months, like fruit and nuts, but also, as Ray said, "It's your birthday; have some cake."

Let's talk about chocolate cake. When I was a child, chocolate cake was a treat. My mom would make me a chocolate cake on my birthday, and we'd all feast. But I didn't have chocolate cake every week or even every month—I had it on my birthday, and maybe a couple other times a year at other birthday celebrations, and maybe once at a restaurant. Mom baked a few chocolate cakes a year.

That's not the way it was in my fat adult life. Chocolate cake was there whenever I wanted it, and it was there to make me want it. When I would go to the airport, which was almost every week, I'd get a cup of coffee at Starbucks and maybe a "muffin" for "breakfast." A triple chocolate "muffin" with chocolate chips in it. What the fucking fuck? That's a muffin like bin Laden was a protester. Starbucks sells chocolate cake with more calories than my mom's birthday chocolate cake, and they sell it for breakfast. When I ate my mom's chocolate cake it was at a little party and we'd all be wearing little hats, and we'd take a bite and praise my mom for her baking and think about the cake and enjoy it and then have another piece or maybe two and say, "Oh, I ate too much." The Starbucks chocolate cake? I'd eat that while talking on the phone at the airport. It was nothing. It wasn't an event. It was just "breakfast." Get something in my stomach to get me through the flight to L.A., where I would walk into a meeting to find more muffins and bagels and cream cheese and Yoplait, which is yogurt like a Snickers bar is a peanut, and yogurt isn't good for you to begin with. So I had come home: I ate my birthday chocolate cake with CrayRay in celebration, just like I'd eaten my mom's chocolate cake. Except this time wasn't as good; fucking vegans.

One of the many nonintuitive—well, just bug-nutty crazy— things about my new way of eating is it got me excited about food that I'd been eating and not caring about. I hadn't been excited about chocolate cake in decades. Why would I be—I was having it while walking around in airports. It wasn't an event.

When I was a child, our family went out to eat regularly, but not often. This was when Roquefort dressing was fifty cents extra and my mom got it because it was a big treat and she liked "exotic" foods. Maybe once every month or so, we'd go out for steak. That was a big deal. The food we ate at home at this time would make CrayRay crazier, but the restaurant food, although not quite Rare and Appropriate, at least wasn't constant.

As I grew up and got more successful, I could afford to eat out at really nice places. Business meetings in cities where I was working would be held at steak houses, where the blue cheese dressing didn't cost a penny extra and you could put it on your steak. With the exception of Skyline Chili in Cincinnati and Durgin-Park in Boston, there was no restaurant that was a rare treat for me. They even had Krispy Kreme doughnuts in Vegas, and the owner of the shop would bring them backstage for us. I had plenty of money to eat at any restaurant, and I usually didn't need to pay.

Andy Warhol had his NYC artist diet where when someone took you out to supper, you would order the most expensive thing on the menu that you didn't like, push it around on the plate, asked to have it boxed up, and give it to a homeless person. I never did that. I ate everything on the table. The celebration was constant. But as the fat and sickness build up, there's no real joy. It's like having someone lick your genitals twenty-four hours a day, every day . . . okay, bad example.

Now, on the Penn's R&A program, I would be able to look forward to food again. And every two weeks is really often. If I had a birthday party every two weeks, I'd be 1,580 years old, and when I was eating muffins at Starbucks every day, I felt that old. (I know, I know, back off—I've gotten lost here, haven't I? I've conflated the R&A every two weeks with the muffin/chocolate cake at Bucky's every day; the two-week time frame is from the new eating, and the muffin and the feeling sick are from the old eating. I've ended up kinda making the opposite point that I was trying to make. But as fucked-up as it is, it's not nearly as bad as comparing bin Laden to a muffin, and we got by that, didn't we?)

I had chocolate cake on my birthday, and I could stop losing weight. I just had to maintain my weight, which is way harder. It seems that most anyone can lose weight, but keeping the weight off for a couple of years is something only about 1 percent of dieters do. "One Percent" is a term some bikers use. I had a buddy who used to be a really bad guy, who got a tattoo in prison, strictly jailhouse, that read "1%." It supposedly comes from a statement made a long while ago by the American Motorcycle Association that 99 percent of motorcyclists were law-abiding citizens. So those who prided themselves on being outlaws started calling themselves "one percenters." I was just about to suggest that we co-opt that term for people who live outside the law of SAD and keep the weight off and stay healthy for years after losing it. As I began to type that, I realized that I was suggesting taking something away from people who pride themselves on being outlaw bikers and going to prison. I have no problem pissing off magicians and ventriloquists, but outlaw bikers . . . I think we should respectfully let them have that term, so I'll say that I hoped my Fuhrburger with the added two-week rule would put me in the vast minority. How's that?

I'll write about my daily eating elsewhere. I'm writing about R&A here. So the rule I set up for myself was that I'd go at least fourteen days between breaks in the Fuhrman diet, and I would try to keep that to one meal, which I loosely defined as four hours. I also added to that, half jokingly, that I would only do my R&A at really expensive restaurants, and when someone else was paying.

March 20 was two weeks out from my chocolate cake and the first day the Penn rules would allow Rare and Appropriate, but I waited three weeks more. I didn't do my next R&A until April 10. I hope this means I've learned a little bit about how to control myself. Knowing that I could have "anything I wanted" made it much easier to eat the way I *really* wanted to. Five weeks was easy, because those were five weeks of maintenance eating, not eating to lose weight. Finally the day came that seemed right. A couple of friends were going with EZ and me to see Diana Ross, and they invited us out to dinner. It was a nice expensive place, and I knew they were paying. Oh boy, time to Rare and Appropriate all over their asses.

I had no idea what to expect. I had heard stories from my hippie friends about not eating meat for a while and then having a taste of hamburger, which made their guts go nutty. Just disgusting. You could fit everything I know about the microbiome into a bacterium, but I was afraid that all the cooties that digested animal products for me were dead and gone, and I'd wind up clutching my guts and running to the restroom. CrayRay told me to be careful on this first R&A and not go too crazy. I told CrayRay to go fuck himself.

I was afraid of getting sick, but that didn't stop me. I was even more afraid of not getting sick and loving the food. I was more afraid that I'd like it, feel great, and realize what I'd been missing, and then never be able to go back to the diet. If I got sick, the night would suck, and if I loved it, the night would suck. I was celebrating eating well by eating badly . . . but it had been five weeks, and someone else was paying.

When I said CrayRay could fuck himself, I meant it. I ate everything that night. Everything. I ate fried calamari. I'd had nothing fried for five months, not even one taste of a freedom fry, but I started pounding down the breaded, greasy, rubber-band *Star Trek: The Appetizer* wonder that is squid. It was good. I couldn't wait to get my mouth around bread and butter. I'd had no bread or anything like bread and no butter or anything like butter for five months, and it was good. Fresh hot bread with creamy butter at the right temperature is the best. I put the butter on thick and yellow, without guilt. There was a basket of assorted breads, and I had to try them all. Well, "try" didn't enter into it—I ate them all. My friends kept asking me what it was like, and I kept saying "Good." I was pounding in the food, eating like a freak, but I was distracted by what I was feeling. I wasn't feeling that I had to rush to the restroom, but I also wasn't feeling feasting heaven. I was feeling okay, and nothing could have shocked me more. Hey there, cheese—let's eat all of you. Yum. There were mussels in garlic butter sauce with that nice bread to dip into the butter, but I buttered the bread before sticking it into the butter because that's the kind of guy

I am. I had a superfancy restaurant bacon cheeseburger, because that was the last thing I'd craved when I still had cravings. I put mayo and ketchup on that bad boy, and I had really salty French fries swimming in sugary ketchup. The closest thing I had to health food was a chickpea side dish, but even those were deep-fried. Worried that I might be skimping on the animal fat, salt, and more fat and salt, I had paté and salty pickles. It was all good. Then it was time for dessert, and I had a big gooey chocolate dish with caramel and a molten center. I ate a lot of food. It was amazing how much I ate, but what's more amazing was that this was about what I would have eaten before I started this diet, or if I wasn't being careful on any other diet. 2014 Penn would not have been appalled. This is what I would have eaten, and it didn't taste any better than it had tasted when I was fat. It didn't taste any worse. I wasn't disgusted by all the fat and sugar. The animal products didn't seem dirty and awful. It just seemed the same.

It shocked me how normal it felt, and I was only slightly haunted by how sick I was going to be. How I would be regretting eating like a pig. CrayRay had told me to be careful. He had said my guts might not be able to handle this, and I was ignoring CrayRay and eating another taste of someone else's dessert. I kept being shocked that nothing was shocking. It was neither good nor bad—I was just eating. The check came, and I didn't pay a cent. I didn't even offer to pay the tip. My costs would all come later as this hit my guts.

We headed over to Diana Ross's show, and I kept worrying about getting sick and having to leave. My mouth had written a check that my intestines were about to default on. I had starved all my fat-fuck allies in my microbiome, and all that were left were the wimpy veg eaters. I knew there would be hell to pay—I just hoped it wouldn't be too embarrassing. I enjoyed the show. Diana Ross didn't embarrass herself, either.

My first R&A turned out to be better in a way I couldn't have imagined. The food didn't taste better than it would have tasted when consuming that shit was chronic; it was just about the same. I didn't get sick, and it wasn't sickening to me. It was just food. Food that I don't usually eat. What I couldn't have predicted was nothing: no big deal. This was the best news possible. I was dancing. Bob Dylan once said he wanted to play guitar without tricks. I've thought about that a lot. If a musician is really good, you have no idea how good he or she is. They play what is right for the music, no more and no less. If what is right is a Johnny Cash open-chord strum, he or she plays that, and if the song requires a moment of Van Halen, he or she plays that. The skill is in service to the art. Teller and I try to do magic without tricks. If you take that at the surface level, I hope we've failed, but at a deeper level it's what we're going for. There should be an ease and clarity to anything that's real and from the heart. Things that are true shouldn't have tricks. Can we do magic tricks without showbiz tricks? That's what we're trying for.

Diana Ross was great. She can sing. She was never working too hard to hit the notes and sell the song. She had real bona fide hits, and she sang them perfectly. She wasn't desperate, she wasn't cloying; she was a pro. She sang her Motown without tricks (except for maybe when she told us to "follow your dreams" as an afterthought). As Supreme as she was, I was more blown away by CrayRay. As I stood in the audience dancing, I was thinking about how "follow your dreams" seems like irresponsible advice. Should I really have a sex orgy with all the MILFs at my daughter's school in the middle of Disney's Main Street Electrical Parade while the original Iron Butterfly plays "In-A-Gadda-Da-Vida" live while Lord Buckley dances naked in a derby? Maybe that is a good idea, but the important thing is that I was thinking about that and not about food in either a positive or a negative way. It's possible that CrayRay had gotten me to diet without tricks. I wasn't dieting at all. I was simply eating. I ate good food to be healthy most of the time, and then once in a while, when it was Rare and Appropriate—meaning someone else was paying—I'd eat food that was more decadent. When the song required it, I could bang out some three-chord rock 'n' roll, but that wasn't all I was able to play.

CrayRay was wrong about one thing—my gut handled the food fine. The huge influx of salt, fat, and sugar might have been microbiome Woodstock, but it sure wasn't Katrina. I felt better after eating that expensive SAD meal, post-CrayRay, than I would have when I was eating like that chronically. When I ate like that all the time, far from being used to it, I felt awful after every big meal, and that meant *every* meal. I felt sluggish and shitty. How surprising that eating this meal when I was out of practice would feel better than when I was a professional fat fuck. I felt a little overfull and little yecch, but not that bad. The salt fucked up my mouth a bit. My mouth didn't seem fresh and wholesome. I could feel the salt on the membranes flowing inside me. I was really thirsty, but not in a panicked way. That was the downside of the meal, but I was more worried about the upside—and, as it turned out, that was fine, too. There was no temptation to eat like that the rest of the night or the next day. One drink was not too many. I didn't fall off the wagon. It was beyond perfect—it was just kind of nothing. I got home and chatted with CrayRay about it a lot. I was over-the-moon happy. He had predicted all sorts of digestion problems, but it was all fine, and the next day there was no real weight change—just the usual pound or so fluctuation. Even my blood pressure didn't spike. I had some trouble falling asleep because my guts were rumbling a bit, but they weren't going crazy. I felt fine. Wow, Bob Dylan and CrayRay, working together.

Afterward, the every-two-week plan remained in effect, but two weeks after Diana, nothing came up. A whole month went by before my buddy Mac King called and said he wanted to take me out to supper. Maybe this was becoming a thing. Since people knew that my going out for Rare and Appropriate was going to be rare, they wanted to be part of it. Mac asked if he could take me to supper when I wanted to be off Fuhrman, and he would pay. Good thinking. Mac is the best act in Vegas. He does an afternoon show at Harrah's that is the best comedy magic show I've ever seen. Most comedy magic shows aren't really funny and don't really have good magic. His comedy magic show would hold up without tricks as a comedy show and without jokes as a magic show. Mac is good. Mac is also a good friend. Mac was the first of us to slide into crazy diet world. Mac was never a fat fuck, but Mac had high cholesterol. He read *The China Study* by T. Colin Campbell and Thomas M. Campbell II and stopped all animal products. We made fun of him, and I thought he wasn't getting enough protein. I worried about his weight loss and his health while I was a fat fuck. I think Mac coined the phrase "unethical vegan" for how he'd just pick bacon off the salad and then eat it. Animal products weren't magic—he just didn't eat them. Mac was the first of us to get healthy with diet, but we kind of didn't notice it until CrayRay came into our lives. Now Mac wanted us to go out together and eat a lot of the kind of food we now ate only rarely.

I considered changing my rule to once-a-month R&A, but it seemed like having the rule be *at least* two weeks and then often a month was fine. Mac and I made a date. Our family had just bought a new house in the fancy section of Vegas over by Mac's place, and there was a really nice steak house where he knew the owners and stuff. He would pay, and we would eat like pigs.

I have sent a lot of customers to Mac's show. If you're in Vegas and you want to see a great show in the afternoon, go see him, and please tell him I sent you. I need to send a lot of business his way just to make up for what I ate on Mac's dime that Rare and Appropriate night in May. I had foie gras, steak tartare, bread and butter, a shellfish platter, a tomahawk steak, mac and cheese waffles, and a twice-baked potato. Of course I left room for dessert, which was an apple tart, ice cream, fancy-ass-rich-person doughnuts with dipping sauce, and cheesecake (I couldn't make up my mind). I believe there wasn't one mouthful I ate that would have been part of my usual diet. Animal products, salt, fat, oil, refined grains—all of it. My mouth dried out and tasted awful from the salt. I was a little sluggish, but it was fine. It wasn't a thing in either direction. Two professional magicians dieting without tricks. CrayRay had said months before that it was fine to have Thanksgiving dinner, and when you say, "I'm not going to eat for days after this," just don't. So the day after the Mac feast I didn't eat until suppertime, and then very lightly. It wasn't a big deal to me, but I wasn't around when his AmEx bill came in.

When I instated my R&A plan, I also told our manager, the long-suffering Glenn, that my change in diet would not affect me professionally in any way. In order to sell our live Vegas show, we have to go on TV. This means I do crazy shit like *The Celebrity Apprentice* and *Celebrity Wife Swap*. My buddy Rob Pike observed that anytime a field of science had the word "science" in it, it wasn't science: "computer science," "social science"—you get the idea. That idea is also absolutely true for the word "celebrity." If a TV show has "celebrity" in the title, there won't be a real celebrity to be found. Remember, it wasn't *The Celebrity Beatles at Shea Stadium*. It's not *The Celebrity Jay Z Show* or *All-Celebrity Avengers*. Because I'm not much of a celebrity, I go on celebrity shows all the time. I used to think that to sell tickets to our little magic show I had to go on TV and do magic. That's just not true. It doesn't seem to matter what I do on TV. Donald Trump likes to claim that without his having had me on his TV show, Penn & Teller would be nothing. He is, of course, wrong. First of all, it wasn't his fucking show. We were both actors on an NBC show—it wasn't his show. And I wasn't on the show to get a job from him. He had no job to offer me, I wasn't looking for a job, and he didn't fire me, because I wasn't working for him. None of that really happened, and everyone in America except Trump, that deluded motherfucker with hair that looks like cotton candy made of piss, knows that. I really like Trump a lot. I do—but I like him as a coworker, not as a boss or a president. I guess I kinda sorta worked for him when he maybe kinda sorta owned an Atlantic City casino that P&T worked at—but then that joint went bankrupt on his watch.

All that being said (and said over and over—I kind of say that shit every chance I get), Trump was right about the big picture. *The Celebrity Apprentice* sold more tickets to Penn & Teller than anything else we've done. It's true that we were already in the Penn & Teller Theater and had been running successfully before Trump and I did that show together, but those "celebrity" shows sure helped a lot.

There are a lot of "celebrity" cooking shows, so I have to go on those, too. And when I was asked to be a judge or a contestant on a cooking show, I didn't want to do that as a nutritarian. If a TV show was serving SAD or I was asked to cook SAD, that is what I would eat. And anything that came through the P&T office would be automatically off the diet—an automatic R&A without a two-week timer running.

I've used that "automatic R&A without a two-week timer running" only once, and it was seven weeks after my last R&A, so I didn't really need the "celebrity" dispensation. When we were getting our big return to Broadway together, I had to fly to London for a day to do a TV show over there and then back to NYC to do Bobby Flay and Jimmy Fallon, and then back to Vegas the next day. Jimmy Fallon tore his finger off, so I just did Bobby Flay. I was excited. Even though the time frame put me in R&A territory, I liked that it was a special "celebrity" feast. I was going to judge, which is the best way to be on these cooking shows. If you're ever given a choice, be a judge and not a contestant. These shows are not real, but by the time you get to being judged, it's very hard to remember that. The flop sweat and anxiety are very real.

I got to the Bobby Flay set and decided that it wasn't just when I was on camera but also all the time backstage that I was off the healthy clock. In my trailer was muffin cake, but it didn't seem great, so I didn't have any. In the green room there was chocolate. Lots of chocolate. There were M&Ms, which I love, and also really fancy chocolate, which I also love. I grabbed a handful of M&Ms, my first in over six months, and they were . . . waxy and cloying, with a really bad aftertaste. What the fucking fuck? CrayRay had fucked me so deep and hard that he'd ruined me for M&Ms. I tried the fancy, expensive chocolate and it was okay, but it was too sweet, and this was the dark shit. I liked my plain cocoa on fruit better. There was a cheese platter, and that just tasted greasy and spoiled. I'm exaggerating here. It wasn't disgusting, it just wasn't great. I was tasting forbidden fruit, and it wasn't that big a deal. It just wasn't good. It was vaguely disappointing, like when I found out that gay sex was all stuff I'd done with women, just done with a guy. There was nothing special. This food was all good; it's nice to eat—but I enjoyed my straight diet better.

I went out to judge the food and found it was pasta, which I've missed, and soup, which I love. The pasta tasted like oil and salt to me. That's nice, but it didn't blow me away. I then found out that I wasn't going to get to judge the round where Bobby Flay made steak. What the fucking fuck? I begged, so they slipped me a perfect steak with a nice cheese sauce, along with some potato thing. Just great. And I ate that and liked it. I liked it fine, but it wasn't magic. I sure didn't want any more of it. Just to show that I was still me, I went to craft services and grabbed some good old plain Lay's potato chips—and ate them the way they should be eaten, shoving as many as possible in my mouth at once, and . . . they just tasted salty and slightly spoiled. It was so easy to go back to my Fuhrburger diet. So easy. CrayRay had given me all the skills, and they were embedded so deep in me that I could just live my life. No obsessing over food, no deals with myself, no cheating—I was just healthy.

When the P&T Broadway run first started, I had one accidental R&A. It's the only one I've had that I didn't plan in advance. Our family went out to a restaurant that EZ loves, one with an antipasto bar and a lot of vegetables. The menu was filled with vegan soups, and it seemed like maybe I could just order. I ordered vegan soup and beets, and what came was full of salt and oil. It was clearly not the Fuhrburger way. I didn't want to send it back and get something different full of server hate-spit. I realized it had been more than two weeks since my last R&A and it would be easy to wait another two weeks after this, so I ate food that was okay but not too decadent, and used up an R&A. This was a restaurant that featured chocolate-covered peanut brittle as a post-dessert dessert (what have we become?), so I had handfuls of that on the way out and called it an R&A meal.

Penn & Teller were on Broadway for six weeks (and did very well, thank you very much—check out the *New York Times* write-ups). Being in New York, I needed a couple of days to eat food that was dictated not by CrayRay but by Original Ray.

The first R&A in NYC was going to be at Katz's Deli. I would have gone to Carnegie Deli in Midtown, but they were closed, so I was going to Katz's. Our whole family went downtown. We went up in One World Trade Center and looked at the beautiful view of the city and out at the Statue of Liberty from high up in the new building. I tried to explain to my children why this new building made Daddy a little sad. After that, it was time for a cupcake. I had a nice gooey-frosted fancy-ass chocolate cupcake in the food area of the World Trade Center as my appetizer, and then we were off to Katz's.

I had a lot of pickles, an egg cream, and four cans of Cel-Ray soda to start. I love Cel-Ray. The idea of a sugary soft drink that tastes like celery kills me. It seems like a joke, like blue cheese gum, but it's great. The fact that it tastes like celery doesn't mean it has anything to do with celery—it's just carbonated sugar water. Four cans was enough for the meal, the day, the week, the month, the year, and maybe the rest of my life, but I loved it. Then I had matzo ball soup, and I ate some of EZ's bagel with lox and cream cheese. I had thick, greasy French fries and then the thing I was living for: a nice big corned beef and pastrami on rye with mustard. Just perfect. I wanted to enjoy my NYC deli meal, and I played it up big for my family and friends, how much I was eating and how much I was loving it . . . but it was kinda bullshit. The cravings were gone. CrayRay really had ruined me. I ate the whole sandwich with mustard but not with relish (that joke is just for my wife; she loves that kind of cheesy wordplay shit—just ignore it). The truth is, it seemed like crankcase oil on a salt lick. It was a little disgusting. This is nothing against Katz's—they put out a great product, and you have to try it. They haven't changed—I have. The cheesecake was the same: delicious, but not for me. We went to see a shitty musical, and after that I had some soft-serve ice cream from a street vendor. I didn't really love any of it, and I felt like shit. Not explosive embarrassing shit, but I didn't feel good. Just too full, sluggish, and oversalted. The next day my weight was down three pounds (normal fluctuation) and my BP was really good. One New York deli, even a great one, couldn't fuck me up.

I know a lot about Broadway and NYC, so let's get into areas where I'm really talking out of my ass. That's where I'm at my best. Let me write a little about the microbiome. That's close to my ass. CrayRay sent me a study that said some of the cooties that fuck up your heart and circulatory system are not cooties that are directly in the food. It's not like you eat this fucking crankcase oil and that goes into your heart and clogs it up. The way I understand it (which means "wrong") is that the animal-fat-eating cooties in your microbiome eat the animal fat and then shit (do bacteria shit?) out waste, and it's the bacteria-shit-cooties that fuck up your heart. That's how I understand it. So there's this study that CrayRay sent me that I skimmed and didn't understand, and which I'm not referencing as I write this, that I think showed if they took someone who eats a SAD and gave him a hunk of prime rib and then checked his blood, it was filled with bad cooties, but if they took that same prime rib (well, not the same one—that's really disgusting) and fed it to a person who had been a vegan for a long while, there were many fewer (or maybe none, I don't remember) cooties in the hippie's blood. That's nuts. I didn't make this up, I just misunderstood and misremembered it. The way I understand this (which is not at all) is that if you don't eat meat, you can eat all the meat you want without it hurting you. It's not the meat itself that fucks you, it's the cooties in your guts that eat the meat and shit out heart-cooties that do. After a few months I'd changed my microbiome so that when I did my R&A, there weren't too many meat-cooties to feast in my guts and fuck me up. I could so easily be the science writer for the *New York Times*.

My wife and I love to split a toasted, buttered corn muffin together when we're in NYC. This trip would not have been complete without one of those. Now, "toasted, buttered corn muffin" is yet another phrase for cake, so this would have to be an R&A. A buttered corn muffin is romantic to us, because when we were first married I took EZ to see the greatest live band in the world, NRBQ, when they played near my hometown, and they have a song with the lyric "Terry got a muffin and he buttered it down." Yup—we would have a corn muffin and butter it down. I put aside a day for that a couple of weeks after going to Katz's.

It was the first day I'd done R&A on the same day that I had a P&T show in the evening. I really didn't want to feel sluggish during the show, but I also didn't want to miss a New York City eating day, and I had no more NYC eating days without a show in the evening. That morning I was shooting some web ads for Withings scales, and, after talking about how healthy my diet was, I left the studio in Brooklyn and headed into Manhattan to eat like a pig. This was going to be my street food day. Not gourmet, not expensive, just whatever I would love to eat while walking around Manhattan.

Teller and Jonesy, our piano player, raved about this fancy hot chocolate at Rockefeller Center. I had that. It was fine. Not worth raving about. I went to "Famous" Ray's and had a street slice of pizza. I shook some garlic salt onto it, folded it just right, and ate it. I didn't eat it all. I got sick of it. I let myself have a Sierra Mist lemon-lime soda with it. I had two sips; it was just too fucking sweet. I threw out half the pizza and most of the drink. I walked uptown to Pick-a-Bagel and had an everything bagel with a lot of cream cheese. I also had a decaffeinated coffee, but I put a lot of cream and sugar in. The way I used to drink it when I was a child. The bagel didn't swing just right, so I tried another one, this time without the cream cheese but with a lot of butter. Nope.

I did our Broadway show that night, and it was okay. I might have been a little sluggish, but it was no disaster. After the show, EZ and I went out with Jonesy, the long-suffering Glenn, and some friend of his from high school who couldn't tell a joke to save his fucking life, but didn't know that and so kept telling them. We tried to hip him to his inadequacies, but he wouldn't take a hint. He wouldn't even take, "Hey, you can't tell a fucking joke to save your life."

EZ and I were going to have our toasted corn muffin, but I was already in my R&A window, so I had a lot of diner food that I loved. I had a grilled cheese with bacon, a chocolate milk shake, and a big order of fries, and we each had a corn muffin and we buttered it down. The corn muffin was so big and so sweet and so salty that it was stupid. The next day I went back to Fuhrburger with a smile.

Well, that's not true—it didn't feel like going back, and it didn't feel like it needed a smile. It's just the way things are. There are no tricks. My dear daughter, Mox, asked me to be her Valentine and wanted me to "Please come off your diet and eat candy with me." So, holidays are outside the day-to-day diet and not part of the two-week rule (which is falling away). On Valentine's Day and Halloween, I will have candy. On the Fourth of July I'll have hamburgers and chips. On Thanksgiving I'll have pizza. And on both my children's birthdays I'll have cake, and so should you!

Dr. Fuhrman and Dr. Michael Klaper are big honchos in this eating-better thang. I've met them both, and they're really wonderful men. They know food and health and spend a lot of time talking to people about "cheat days" and going on and off good food. That's a big part of their lives.

I asked Dr. Klaper how often he runs out and has a doughnut or a burger. "Never. I never even think about it." He's been eating well for his whole life. He's wicked healthy and happy. I asked Dr. Fuhrman if he'd ever been to McDonald's in his life.

He said, "Never," and then thought for a moment and said, "I did go once. I wanted a drink of water, and it was the only place around, so I went in and bought a bottle of water." He paused, and then smiled and said, "But I didn't feel good about it." I'm getting there.

FROM TARGET TO BIRTHDAY

CrayRay hadn't seen me in person since Thanksgiving (although he had seen pictures of me). We were going to meet on my birthday, and I was ready for him. I hit my target weight a few days before the target date, so all I had to do was hold the line for a couple of days. On my birthday, CrayRay would move me from "wait loss" to "maintenance." I'd be going from eating one meal a day to eating all day, whenever I wanted. I could also start exercising. And for you old-fashioned people who think counting calories is the way to go, I would be going from about (this is a very rough estimate) a thousand calories a day to (even rougher estimate) about thirty-three hundred calories a day. Adding a couple thousand calories every day would prevent me from losing 0.9 pounds per day the way I had been doing and hold me at my target weight (all numbers except "0.9 pounds per day" are made up—but 0.9 pounds is a couple thousand calories, right?). On my birthday I would start eating like a Fuhrburger pig, but until then I would keep my toes on CrayRay's line and keep my promise to myself.

This was February 28, and as I better fucking know very fucking well, that's my wife's birthday. To celebrate, EZ wanted to take a lot of her friends to the really fancy-ass Caesars hotel buffet and then go see the very attractive and funny Wayne Brady. We had a bunch of seats for the show, but our first stop was the buffet.

There are lots of bullshit studies that say buffets are the worst for healthy eating. To get your money's worth, you gotta cram a lot of salt, fat, sugar, animal products, and refined grains into your gob. Caesars has a good/bad buffet for that, because there's really good meat and crab and fancy desserts. It was EZ's birthday but it wasn't mine yet, so I had to keep on my program; there would be no "Rare and Appropriate" for me yet.

I created a salad at the Caesars buffet that was great, and I haven't had a version of it since. I didn't use any lettuce. There was no rhythm section to this salad. I put in nothing but cilantro, basil, and onions for my base. They had bowls of those to garnish soup, and I just filled a plate with them like they were the entrée. I laid sliced onions like spaghetti on the bottom. Garnishes were the main course. They were no longer twenty feet from stardom, they were my supper. I had a huge plate of cilantro, basil, and onions, and then added a few radishes, carrots, and a lot of really hot peppers. Just the smell of this salad made my eyes water. I piled up the plate with it.

Robin Leach, the *Lifestyles of the Rich and Famous* guy, is a friend of ours, and he loves my wife. He was at Caesars for her birthday party. He was pretty shocked by my weight loss; he's a journalist, so he asked me how I lost all the weight. I told him I had just a touch of Ebola, just right there in the back of the throat, and it took the weight off like crazy. He patronized me with a chuckle and then asked again. I dodged again. He pushed, I pushed back. He pushed again, I pushed back again. I wasn't giving up the info. Not yet. Not until I saw CrayRay.

So Robin observed and counted what I ate and wrote it down. I had four huge plates of this psycho aromatic garnish salad. My only dressing was vinegar, and I loved it. It was Wayne Brady's show and not mine, so I didn't have to worry about being light-headed. I didn't need rice or potatoes or glucose pills. I could just eat my Caesars psycho salad.

By that time, I had decided to write this book about my nutty weight loss, so I thought this salad would be my first recipe. That was my plan. So I took a picture and kind of kept it in my head. But we haven't been able to re-create it at home. Maybe my wife doesn't believe me when I tell her how many raw onions I had, or maybe you just can't get a bowl of cilantro. Maybe we chicken out and sneak in lettuce. I don't know, but I loved this salad, and I haven't had it since.

My weight was down even more the next day. Now I was at 229.1. My target was 229, so I guess you could say I hadn't hit it. But targeting 229 when you're at 304 and hitting it within a tenth of a pound seems like an achievement on par with the NASA guys hitting Pluto. I was pretty fucking proud of myself.

But it wasn't without cost. I'd gone to all salads for a few days to make sure I hit my goal, and that turned out to be a little stupid. Actually, it was way stupid. During the show my light-headedness crossed over into fainting territory. Like, woozy and unsure on my feet. I very nearly lost consciousness during the show. That was really stupid. Also, EZ noticed that I started to smell bad. I went into that Atkins ketosis stink. The whole CrayRay plan is supposed to avoid ketosis, but my body had decided to use ketone bodies for energy instead of glucose. I have no idea what that means, but EZ said I stank, and she didn't like it. After the show I had to catch a charter plane to L.A., so EZ ordered me brown rice, corn, and potatoes from room service to get some starch in me for the flight. I needed to stop breathing out nail polish remover and falling over.

It was a busy day in L.A. We were doing a reality show called *I Can Do That* where we had to teach Joe Jonas and Ciara to do magic. They were wonderful to work with. You get less credit for being skinny when you're around young pop stars, but I liked working with them. We taught them magic, and they were great, but our team lost. I also lost on *Dancing with the Stars, Rachael vs. Guy, Celebrity Chopped, The Celebrity Apprentice,* and *All-Star Celebrity Apprentice.* I lost on all of those. But I won on (celebrity) *Jeopardy!.* Let's think about this: I lost on every show that was subjective, where politics were involved, and I won on the one show that was purely objective. The one where sucking up and backstabbing don't help. So fuck Donald Trump in the neck.

I woke up on March 5, 2015, sixty years old and thinner than I'd been since I was thirty. We'd been flying every day to L.A. to do TV, and then back to Vegas to do our show, with some corporate shows thrown in. We were also meeting with our fellow producers about our American version of *Penn & Teller: Fool Us.* It was a hectic time, and being thinner made it a lot easier. I didn't have to drag that extra hundred pounds back and forth across state lines.

My son, Zolten, had to recite a poem at school. I suggested "Howl," but that was vetoed by EZ and the teacher. I guess they figured Z hadn't seen the greatest minds of his generation destroyed by madness yet. I don't think he's ever really even dragged himself through the Negro streets at dawn looking for an angry fix. So he went with "The Road Not Taken," which is a more depressing poem than "Howl." I practiced it with him, and then we sent him to school in a uniform to recite a poem about how individuality and choices didn't matter. I still contend we would have been better off having him recite that assholes are holy.

I weighed myself on my birthday, and I was at 228.9. So I made it: 229 pounds by my birthday was the goal. I was on the NASA of diets, and that night I was going to see CrayRay.

If you have to turn sixty and weigh 229 pounds, you might as well do it with David Hasselhoff and Kendra and her Wilkinsons, so Teller and I were on the set of *Sharknado 3*. It was cold, in the middle of nowhere, and there were no sharks or tornadoes—let alone sharknadoes—but we were cruisin' with the Hoff, so it was okay. At the end of the shoot, the production was nice enough to bring out a big old birthday cake for me, with candles and everything. They all sang "Happy Birthday," including the Hoff and Kendra. I was a little worried about how I was going to not eat cake without insulting people, and then the guy who was carrying the cake tripped and dropped the whole thing upside down in the mud. Instead of having to be awkward, I got to be gracious.

I went from there to meet a bunch of friends at Real Food Daily, and among those friends was CrayRay himself. This was it. This would be our first meeting since the diet started. It was kind of a big hairy deal. We shook hands and hugged, and then he just kind of looked at me and beamed all over. We were both close to crying, but since we were in a trendy vegan restaurant in Hollywood, we had to maintain some dignity. We were jumping out of our skins with excitement. It's been rare in my life to set out to do something and then do it. No turns, no alibis, no redefined or refined goals, no explanations, no shit! We did it.

We sat down, and I had two bowls of food that was completely acceptable when I was losing. I wouldn't break out of the diet until we got back to the room. We had a chocolate cake (vegan for no reason) and then fruit. CrayRay watched like a proud dad as I had my first piece of fruit in three months. I'd had some little pieces of cut-up strawberries in a salad, or cut-up raspberries, but no bite-into-it fruit.

No real fruit. But now I had dragon fruit. I'd never had that. It was like they invented new fruit while I was away. Think back on when I had corn for the first time after two weeks of potatoes. Could you understand how sweet and great it was? Now I was having food that really is sweet. Even if you're addicted to sugar, fat, and salt, fruit is pretty fucking close to candy. I was just stuffing my face with fruit. I kept looking over at CrayRay like he'd just told me to fuck his hot wife and I wanted to keep making sure it was okay. I expected him to say, "Okay, Penn, let's not go nuts," at any moment. Do you know how many times that's been said to me, in how many situations? But he didn't. He was helping me cut it up. "Try this." "Isn't that good?" I couldn't believe how good fruit was.

"And I can have all I want of this, anytime I want?"

"Sure. You're at your target weight; you can't really go back up eating fruit."

CrayRay insisted I have cake because my birthday was Rare and Appropriate, but it wasn't as good as the fruit. It was too fucking greasy, but the thought was good.

There was a lot to celebrate. We'd gotten another season of our TV show, our Vegas show was breaking records, we had a few national TV shows, and my movie was fully funded and close to done. I could even have been celebrating that I looked so much better and fit into size 36 jeans with room to spare, but none of that mattered; I was really celebrating not feeling like shit. I was celebrating that if I managed to avoid getting hit by a truck or pissing off Teller, I might live to see my children graduate (or at least be socially promoted) from high school. By getting off the blood pressure drugs, I might even live to see them get let down by the college of their choice.

It was really CrayRay's night. He strutted around our hotel suite, the man with the plan. He sat in a chair, and many of my friends gathered at his feet. He told NASA stories and science stories, but mostly he talked about food and health, and I think before he was done about a dozen people from my birthday signed up with him. They all ended up doing great.

Thanks, CrayRay.

YOU SAY IT'S YOUR BIRTHDAY?
WELL, IT'S MY SKINNY
BIRTHDAY, TOO, YEAH

Birthdays don't mean jack shit to me, but this one was the big six-oh, and CrayRay and I had tied it to my weight loss. We had accomplished something that I would have thought impossible just four months earlier. I was off most of my blood pressure meds, and all twelve of my Penn & Teller suits were being retailored. There were meetings at the Rio and in TV studios about how to advertise a show in which one of the stars looked so different. It was like trying to sell the Three Stooges as the same act, even though Curly was now Shemp. Except I looked less like Fat-Fuck Penn than Shemp looked like Curly. People didn't recognize me when I went out in public. Any cheesy magic joke you want to make, like the title of this book, was true—I had made one-third of me, over a hundred pounds, magically disappear. I had become invisible.

EZ did an amazing job with my party. While I was doing a little more shooting with Joe and Ciara for *I Can Do That*, she was over at the venue setting things up and working with the chefs. We had invited almost a hundred friends, a friend for every pound I dropped. We had decided to do it at Brookledge.

Erika Larsen is pure magic. Her dad and uncle started the Magic Castle in Hollywood, and if Erika doesn't know you, you ain't in magic. Her mom, Irene, is Siegfried's best friend, and I've watched them tell dirty jokes to each other in German. How did I know they were dirty? I know both of them. Her daughter, Libby, looks so exactly like Erika that she seems less like a daughter and more like a time-traveling experiment that went very, very well. Libby is often the assistant at the Magic Castle. The Larsens are magic.

They all live at a place called Brookledge. It's in Hollywood, and it's pure Hollywood. It's sexier than the Playboy Mansion, with pools and grottoes and plants and trees and landscaping and garden gnomes and no Cosby. It's unstuck in time. In the Larsen backyard, it could be the swinging '60s with the Carson writers hanging out with magicians, or it could be the twenty-first century with a former fat-fuck Vegas magician's birthday party. EZ and Erika had the whole backyard decked out with banquet tables.

Brookledge is more than just Erika, Irene, and Libby's backyard; it's also the most far-out theater in all of L.A. There's a little ninety-seat room where Erika does the Brookledge Follies: Puddles Pity Party, the Amazing Johnathan, Mac King, Two-Headed Dog, Rob Zabrecky, and Eugene Burger have all played there. It's the best place to see a show, and they have the best shows. It's a salon in Paris, except it's funny. For my birthday show, we set up Piff the Magic Dragon and Billy the Mime.

CrayRay and I had gone back and forth on the menu. CrayRay suggested we serve all the food I used to love—steaks and fried food, grease and salt—and I'd meet with all my friends, eat like a pig, and throw up. He thought it would be "good for the book." I liked that idea. I'm not beyond doing a stunt like that to have something to write about, but . . . the more I thought about it, the more it seemed forced. The cravings for that food were gone, and I really wanted to see my friends. I guess I don't have to explain this too much. It's possible you can understand that I didn't want to puke my guts out on my birthday.

I finally decided on a really fancy meal that was completely Fuhrburger, full-blown nutritarian. This wouldn't be the limited-calorie diet I'd been eating the past few months, this would be the way I was going to eat for the rest of my life. We'd call it "Penn's Future Favorite Foods." Yeah, my friends would have to eat no animal products, no refined grains, and very low salt, sugar, and oil, but fuck 'em—it was my birthday.

EZ had trouble finding chefs. L.A. is crawling with vegan chefs, but I'm not a vegan. All the vegan chefs use tons of oil, salt, and sugar. There were plenty of gluten-free and paleo chefs, but I was crazier than all of them put together. The diet I'd chosen was not an L.A. fad; it was kind of science-y and shit.

EZ talked to Jet Tila, but he was scared to give it a try. He turned us on to Taji Marie, a well-known L.A. vegan chef, writer, and winner of *Chopped* (which you may recall I lost the celebrity version of). She had never cooked nutritarian, but she had done a lot of stuff that was close, and she was up for a challenge. EZ, CrayRay, and Taji were going to work on a completely healthy feast for all my friends. There would be no alcohol, no drugs, and plenty of food that was purely Fuhrburger. It would answer my friends' question "What the fuck do you eat now?"

I didn't have much to do with it, but I did tell Taji about some of my old favorite foods. I didn't want her to try to fake those dishes with nutritarian ingredients, but I was hopeful she could pick up some of the vibe. It's like writing a song with Jonesy. I bang out some lyrics and then say, "It's kind of a 'Positively 4th Street' vibe." I don't want to rewrite "Positively 4th Street," but I want some of those feelings.

My mom cooked every meal for me when I was growing up, and the food she cooked means comfort to me. She cooked a New England boiled dinner: corned beef and cabbage in a pressure cooker with carrots, beets, onions, parsnips, potatoes—it's a root-vegetable-and-tuber thang with some mustard on the side. All cooked in one pot. She cooked pork in gravy, and macaroni and cheese with real sharp Vermont cheddar and big fat elbow noodles. She made blueberry pies from scratch with blueberries that she picked herself. When my mom died at the age of ninety, her freezer held blueberries she had picked herself. My friend David Greenberger asks, if you have balloons that were blown up by someone you love right before they died, are those happy or sad balloons? Are those freezer blueberries happy or sad? I don't know; I couldn't bring myself to eat them. Mom has been dead for over fifteen years, and it doesn't seem unlikely that those blueberries are still in the freezer. I'm afraid to ask Chris, who lives there now and takes care of the place. I don't want to know. My mom also made tuna dip. Yeah, tuna dip. It was cans of tuna fish mashed up with cream cheese, and you dipped crackers into it. You know, that Kraft food from the '60s that people put on Facebook with " 'Like' if you remember this," and it's supposed to be disgusting. My mom served a lot of that, and it was wonderful. "Click 'Like' and go fuck yourself."

Of all the food my mom served, the dish I remember the best (maybe because it's the only one I can make) is one she called "Penn's Favorite Salad." It's not "salad" in the modern sense but in the '60s way, where things with marshmallow and lime Jell-O could be called "salad" with a straight face. Kind of like the way things with a slab of greasy salmon on them can be called "salad" now. "Salad" is a nutty word.

"Penn's Favorite Salad" is orange Jell-O, made with some of the water replaced by the strained juice from a can of crushed pineapple.

The pineapple-juice-infused orange Jell-O sits in the fridge until it hits the jiggle consistency of a Russ Meyer close-up. In the meantime, you grate carrots (grate, motherfucker, not shred; this salad is all about texture). When your Jell-O's jiggle is just right, you mix the drained crushed pineapple and the grated carrots together into a yellow-orange pile of goodness and fold (is that the right word? I don't know cooking) it into the Kitten Natividad–jiggly Jell-O and let it set. Then you need the "stuff that makes it good." Take a little bit of leftover strained pineapple juice and mix it with some Miracle Whip to make it a little less viscous. Add a little food coloring, maybe pink to go with the orange of the Jell-O, and cover the big bowl of Jell-O with the stuff that makes it good.

To the twenty-first-century palate, that's pretty disgusting, but the mouth-feel of grated carrots, crushed pineapple, and Jell-O is amazing. And that weird, tart bite of Miracle Whip makes it really groove. When my mom made it, my dad would always grate the carrots on the grating side of one of those square-silver-sharp-mystic-pyramid things. Dad wanted to do it for me, but he wasn't good at grating, so he'd always catch his knuckles and there would be just a little of his blood in the mix. This was back when we weren't so worried about catching pathogens from blood, back in the days when blood in Jell-O was fine and I was eating animal products like my dad's finger flesh. I would have a big bowl of this stuff for dessert and then another for breakfast the next morning. I love it.

I told Taji all about my love of Mom's Jell-O and asked her to try to be inspired by that. She came up with "Grilled Pineapple and Shaved Carrot Salad with Tamarind-Lime Drizzle." She used pineapple, multicolored carrots, tamarind paste, lime, mint, just a smidgen of olive oil, and toasted coconut to give me a modern version of the Kraft delight. (All the recipes from the party are in another chapter.) With my new palate, it was pretty great.

I love tacos, too, so we had tacos with jackfruit that were as good as any pulled-pork taco I'd ever had.

I've realized since the party that there really isn't any reason to try to catch the vibe of foods that I used to love. It's better to just create new comfort food. As EZ kept cooking Fuhrburger dishes, some of them stuck. Now instead of grilled cheese and tomato soup, I crave Fuhrburger's pea soup with dill. It makes me feel all warm and cozy, and doesn't make me feel like my mouth is drying out and my stomach is filled with putty.

The problem with big parties like this is they are filled with my friends. I wanted to talk to everyone there, but because there were so many people, I didn't get to talk to any of them very much. Lawrence O'Donnell Jr., my buddy and MSNBC host, pleased everyone by sticking both his hands all the way down the front of my pants, ostensibly to demonstrate how loose my 36-inch-waist pants were. Eddie Gorodetsky, the funniest writer in the world, shook my hand while handing me a ten-dollar bill, winked, and said, "Buy yourself something nice, and don't tell your grandmother." Tim Jenison, the star of *Tim's Vermeer*, was there; Rif and Pete from *Director's Cut* were there; as were all sorts of magicians, musicians, poets, artists, and people I love. Yeah, it was my birthday, and I'd just lost all this weight, but it wasn't long before I realized that CrayRay was the star. Me, I was proof of concept. People were fighting to get to talk to him. All sorts of people wanted to become CroNuts. He was signing people up like crazy.

When we all piled into the little theater for the entertainment, my mother-in-law rushed to get the seat next to Lawrence O'Donnell— she was so happy to bathe in the aura of a bona fide progressive/liberal TV star in this wasteland of libertarians and anarchists.

Libby welcomed everyone to her home and introduced me. I walked onstage all skinny and shit and introduced CrayRay, who brought down the house explaining how he killed the fat fuck who had eaten me. And then Piff the Magic Dragon took the stage.

Way back before Piff was a Magic Dragon, before he did *Penn & Teller: Fool Us* or *America's Got* [*sic*] *Talent* and moved to Vegas, while he was still an evangelical Christian back in England (yeah, they have those in England), he used to do gospel magic. He used magic tricks to spread the word of Jesus Christ. Piff knows I love gospel magic. I love an overextended metaphor. I love straining a magic trick to make it fit didactic patter (the story of Penn & Teller). He did a gospel magic trick for me. Instead of patter, Piff used a piece of modern, heartfelt, really earnest Christian music. Really earnest, sincere Christian music, and people were laughing their asses off. Some of us, though, were laughing in a different way, glancing back over our shoulders. The superstar producer who had produced the music Piff was having fun with was sitting in the audience. He's a friend of mine. He's not an atheist, and he was watching a magic dragon have some fun with his masterpiece while atheists guffawed. If Piff had known, he would have still done it. Not all my friends are atheists, but all my friends can take a joke. That being said, after the show I sure enjoyed telling Piff who that gentleman in the corner was. You don't often get to see a magic dragon blush.

Piff was followed by Billy the Mime. I've seen a lot of great acts and shows in my life, but I've never seen anyone better than Billy. Billy the Mime is Steven Banks. I met Steven in 1979. He went to San Francisco on his honeymoon and came to see us in the Asparagus Valley Cultural Society. He hung around to meet me after the show (instead of banging his wife, but they've been married almost forty years now, and he knew at the time they were going to have lots of time for banging). We were amazed that we were both graduates of Ringling Bros. and Barnum & Bailey Clown College. We both hated drugs and loved the Sex Pistols. We're the same age and have so much in common. We've been friends since that day in Frisco, and Steven has gone on to write for *SpongeBob SquarePants* and bunches of other cartoon shows and plays. He performs college shows, plays in bands, and directs, and it seems he can do anything. He had studied mime, and as far back as I can remember he was talking about doing a mime show for people who hate mime (which is everyone). *Billy the Mime* is that show. Steven performs in classic mime makeup and black tights, and he mimes subjects that mimes usually don't cover.

Here is his set list for my birthday party:

A Romance

JFK, Jr.

World War II

Thomas Jefferson & Sally: A Night at Monticello

A Day with ISIS

Whitney Houston's Last Bath

Priest and Altar Boy

The Unfortunate Magician

The History of Art

Drinks with Bill Cosby

Bobbi Kristina Brown's Last Bath

Clown & Beautiful Woman

You would think just the idea of doing mime about these subjects would be enough to make it a surreally sick humor event. But that's not enough for Billy. He does all the mime perfectly. Every move is perfect and tells the story. But that's still not enough for Billy. It's all filled with heart and love. There's even compassion for the monsters who are represented. It's the most perfectly rounded theater experience: funny, shocking, surprising, tender, thought-provoking, and beautiful.

So, there I was on my birthday. I felt healthy, skinny, and happy. I was surrounded by my friends. I had the best entertainment possible and wonderful food that was going to save my life. A bunch of us then went back to our room, where CrayRay held court.

It was a fuck of a way to turn sixty.

I'd accomplished the short-term goal, and it had been easy. Now I was starting the long-term goal. The hard part. I wanted to stay healthy for the rest of my life.

MY NEW FAVORITE FOODS
BIRTHDAY MENU

APPETIZERS

SAFFRON COCONUT TOMATO SOUP SHOTS
(saffron, cumin, tumeric, fresh tomatoes,
coconut milk, chives, shredded coconut)

I've always liked the idea of shots. I don't drink (we had decaffein-ated tea and coffee and bubbly water for beverages), but the idea of shots appeals to me—big intense mouthfuls, and done. And I love soup. My dad loved soup and taught me to love soup. He also taught me to love ritual jokes. There were certain jokes he did every time the chance came up. Every time my dad had soup, he'd say, "Once I had soup while my nose was running, and I thought I'd never finish." It wouldn't have worked for a shot glass of tomato soup . . . but my dad would still have done it.

EZEKIEL CROSTINI WITH ARTICHOKE LEMON BASIL PESTO AND TOASTED PUMPKIN SEEDS AND CHILI FLAKES

(artichoke hearts, lemon zest, fresh basil, garlic,
nutritional yeast, shaved walnuts, chili flakes)

I hadn't had bread or crackers in five months, so this was quite a treat.

ENDIVE WITH CREAMY CASHEW PUREE & ROASTED GRAPES

(endive, cashews, lemon, nutritional yeast,
purple grapes, balsamic vinegar, chives)

Like a groovy, healthy Caesar salad.

GRILLED ZUCCHINI RIBBON ROLLS WITH ROASTED GARLIC WHITE BEAN PUREE, FRESH BASIL & ZAATAR SPRINKLE

(zucchini, olive oil, white beans, miso, garlic,
basil, thyme, sesame seeds, oregano)

It's hard to get a groove out of garlic without salt, but this sure got me started on that path.

MINI CHIPOTLE JACKFRUIT TACOS WITH AVOCADO CREAM, CILANTRO & JALAPEÑOS

(jackfruit, mini corn tortillas, avocados, lime, cilantro, jalapeños,
chipotle chilies, cumin, tomatoes, onions, garlic, cabbage)

I had never had jackfruit before, but it's better than pork. It's great for mouth-feel and taste. EZ has learned to cook these, and we have them all the time. I could live on them.

MAIN COURSES

WILD MUSHROOM & LENTIL RAGÙ OVER SEARED POLENTA WITH HEIRLOOM TOMATO SALSA CRUDA

(dried and fresh wild mushrooms, tamari, onions, garlic, thyme, lentils, cornmeal, tomatoes, garlic, basil, olive oil, chives)

A little olive oil for taste really makes this swing.

BALSAMIC GRILLED PORTOBELLO MUSHROOMS WITH WHITE BEANS, SLOW ROASTED TOMATOES, AND BASIL & SHAVED FENNEL SALAD SERVED OVER ZUCCHINI NOODLES TOPPED WITH SHAVED WALNUT "PARMESAN"

(mushrooms, balsamic vinegar, rosemary, garlic, white beans, thyme, tomatoes, basil, fennel, chives, zucchini, olive oil, walnuts, nutritional yeast)

Portobello mushrooms with funky walnuts. This is as good as any steak.

INDIAN-SPICED CARROT STEW OVER TOASTED MILLET & SPINACH PILAF TOPPED WITH TOASTED CHICKPEAS, SERVED WITH SPICY MINT-LIME CHUTNEY

(carrots, chickpeas, onions, coconut milk, cumin,
tumeric, garlic, coriander, smoked paprika,
millet, spinach, mint, lime, jalapeños)

I love Indian food, and this be that.

SIDE DISHES

GRILLED PINEAPPLE AND SHAVED CARROT SALAD WITH TAMARIND-LIME DRIZZLE

(pineapple, multicolored carrots, tamarind paste,
lime, mint, olive oil, toasted coconut)

My favorite food was my mom's Jell-O salad with carrots and pine-
apple and Miracle Whip on top. Well, this ain't that, but it's close in
texture and idea. It's not Dylan doing Dylan, but it's better than the
Byrds doing Dylan.

WHOLE WHEAT FLATBREAD WITH SPICED CARROT "BUTTER"

(spelt whole-grain flour, unsweetened almond milk,
cashews, carrots, star anise, coriander, cardamom, dates)

Once again, not having had bread, I ate this like a freak.

TRIPLE GREENS WITH PEANUT-SESAME DRESSING
(broccolini, swiss chard, snap peas, peanuts, tahini,
dates, lime, garlic, jalapeños, cilantro, miso)

I love peanut-sesame anything.

MANGO, AVOCADO, TANGERINE & WATERCRESS
SALAD WITH TOASTED CHICKPEAS
(mango, avocado, tangerines, watercress, chickpeas, smoked
paprika, garlic, cumin, tamarind, lime, chives, dates, olive oil)

*This is one of those things that I wouldn't have even considered taking
a bite of when I was a fat fuck. But now, it's just full of flavors and
textures. And it's food. It's real food. It's what I eat now.*

DESSERTS

COCONUT BROWN RICE PUDDING WITH
SAUTÉED MANGO & TOASTED COCONUT
(brown rice, coconut milk, dates, cinnamon, nutmeg,
mango, shredded coconut, golden raisins)

I've always hated coconut. I loved this.

ROASTED APPLE CRUMBLE WITH COCONUT CREAM

(apples, cinnamon, nutmeg, pear nectar, spelt flour, almonds,
sesame seeds, hemp seeds, flaxseed, coconut milk)

*When I told Taji I wasn't crazy about coconut, she told me I didn't
know what I liked. She was right. I loved this, too.*

It was a perfect meal. It was a healthy feast. More salt, sugar, and oil than I would have every day, but the healthiest feast I ever had. Healthier than any single meal I had ever had before CrayRay.

If you want to taste a few of these things, I asked Taji to give me some of the recipes. Remember, she's a world-class cook, and maybe you're not, but good luck.

CROSTINI WITH ARTICHOKE PESTO
MAKES 24 PIECES

FOR THE BREAD:

6 slices Ezekiel Sprouted Grain bread

2 tablespoons olive oil

1 large garlic clove

FOR THE PESTO:

1 15oz can artichoke hearts

1 small garlic clove

¼ cup pine nuts

1 cup basil leaves

1 teaspoon lemon zest

2 tablespoons brewer's yeast

½ teaspoon ground black pepper

salt to taste

finely minced chives, for garnish

red chili flakes, for garnish

toasted pine nuts, for garnish

Preheat oven to 375 degrees. Brush the bread lightly with olive oil on both sides and place on baking sheet. Toast for 5–10 minutes until just golden. Remove and rub the bread with the garlic clove. Use a two-inch biscuit cutter to cut four rounds out of each slice of bread or cut bread into thin rectangles.

Drain the artichokes and pat very dry. Place in a food processor. Add the garlic, basil leaves, lemon zest, brewer's yeast, and pepper. Pulse until very finely chopped but not puréed.

Dump into a bowl and stir in salt to taste. If desired, stir in more olive oil.

Top each piece of toasted bread with a dollop of the pesto and a sprinkling of chives, chili flakes, and pine nuts. Serve immediately.

GRILLED PINEAPPLE, CARROT & COCONUT SLAW WITH TAMARIND-LIME DRESSING
SERVES 4–6

FOR THE DRESSING:

8 pitted medjool dates

½ cup water

2 limes, zested and juiced

½ cup tamarind paste/concentrate (sometimes sold as "sour soup mix" in Asian stores; look for 100% tamarind as the ingredient)

¼ teaspoon ground nutmeg

½ teaspoon ground cinnamon

3 tablespoons tamari

½ teaspoon granulated garlic

2 tablespoons coconut oil (liquid)

½ teaspoon salt

FOR THE SALAD:

1 pineapple

coconut oil

1 pound multicolored carrots

½ cup shredded unsweetened toasted coconut

½ cup sliced medjool dates

½ cup toasted slivered almonds

Place the dates in a blender with the water. Blend until very smooth, adding just a bit more water as needed. Add the lime zest and juice, tamarind paste, nutmeg, cinnamon, tamari, garlic, coconut oil, and salt. Blend until very smooth.

Heat a grill pan or cast-iron skillet over high heat. Cut the top and bottom off the pineapple, cut away the thick skin, and slice into ½-inch slices. Rub slices lightly with coconut oil. Grill or sear until golden on both sides. Remove and let cool completely.

Cut pineapple pieces into smaller bits and place in a large bowl. Peel and shred the carrots, and add the carrots, coconut, dates, and almonds to the pineapple. Toss with as much dressing as desired. Serve immediately.

MINI JACKFRUIT TACOS WITH AVOCADO
CREAM AND PICKLED SHALLOTS
MAKES ABOUT 24 MINI APPETIZER TACOS

FOR THE JACKFRUIT:

1 can jackfruit in brine (be sure to avoid the jackfruit in syrup)

1 tablespoon coconut oil

1 small white onion, diced

3 garlic cloves, minced

2 tablespoons smoked paprika

2 tablespoons ancho chili powder

1 teaspoon cumin

½ teaspoon cayenne

1 15oz can crushed tomatoes

10 pitted medjool dates

¼ cup brewer's yeast

2 tablespoons apple cider vinegar

2 tablespoons chopped chipotle chili in adobo

2 tablespoons tamari

salt

FOR THE TACOS:

4 shallots

1 cup white vinegar

2 tablespoons honey

1 teaspoon salt

2 avocados

2 tablespoons fresh lime juice

¼ cup cilantro leaves, plus more for garnish

1 garlic clove, grated

2 tablespoons minced jalapeño

3 tablespoons chopped chives

24 mini corn tortillas

Preheat oven to 450 degrees. Drain the jackfruit and rinse very well. Cut away the cores of the jackfruit pieces and discard. Break up the remaining fruit with your hands and spread out on a baking sheet sprayed with oil. Roast for 20–30 minutes or until dried out and golden in places.

Meanwhile, heat a large saucepan over high heat. Add the coconut oil, onions, and garlic.

Reduce heat to medium and cook for 10 minutes until vegetables are soft. Add the smoked paprika, chili powder, cumin, and cayenne. Cook for one minute. Add the tomatoes and dates and cook for 15 minutes, stirring often.

Transfer to a blender. Add the brewer's yeast, vinegar, chipotle, and tamari and blend until smooth. Add salt to taste. Toss the jackfruit with the sauce and keep warm in the saucepan.

Thinly slice the shallots and place in a bowl with the vinegar, honey, and salt. Stir until the honey and salt are dissolved. Cover and refrigerate for at least two hours and up to overnight.

Combine the avocado, lime juice, chopped cilantro, grated garlic, minced jalapeño, and chopped chives. Mash until well combined. Season with salt to taste.

When you're ready to build the tacos, heat the corn tortillas in a dry skillet until very hot. Fill with some of the jackfruit mix and top with the avocado mixture, a few pickled shallots, and some cilantro leaves.

SECTION THREE

EATING PIZZA IS VOTING FOR HILLARY

THE DISAPPEARING MAGICIAN

Friday the thirteenth of March, 2015, I was sitting on a park bench on the banks of the mighty Mississippi. A few benches down, a guy was blowing jazz on a soprano sax. He was good, and I gave him a twenty. A fog lay deep on the water, and Café Du Monde with its great little French-named Dunkin' Munchkins was right behind me with a line of tourists down the block. There was a chill in the air, and a lot of moisture. This sure wasn't Vegas. Penn & Teller would be performing that night at the big theater right outside the French Quarter.

I knew what it meant to walk through the French Quarter when it's crowded. It meant a few pictures every block and a lot of conversation. Siri said that the walk from my hotel to Café Du Monde would take twelve minutes, but I'd allowed thirty minutes for picture taking and talking to the kind folks who had seen me on TV and cared enough to stop me.

I've been appearing on TV regularly for half my life. I made a promise to myself that I wouldn't do any serious TV until I turned thirty. I wasn't asked a lot, but the few times I was, I said no. I thought people with my performer-disease who went on TV before they were thirty went crazy and sometimes died. I didn't want to do that. Also, I knew that if I did go on TV before I was thirty, the first appearance would be kinda easy; Penn & Teller had had years to get the bit together. And the second might be okay, but the third and fourth? At twenty-three years old, I would have been out of material already. So I made this odd arbitrary promise that I wouldn't do TV until I was thirty. Right when I turned thirty I was on *Saturday Night Live* and David Letterman, and started doing Stern like a freak. We never got to be superstars—or ever really stars—but we sure made sub-star pretty solidly.

From that first moment on Letterman, and then the Run-D.M.C. video and *Miami Vice* and so on, I was recognized on the street. I've been out with people who hate being recognized, but I never minded it. The people who recognize me from TV have always been really nice. It's like living in a small town. They just say "Hi, Penn" like they know me from the ice cream social. Did people sometimes stop me in the middle of a conversation to ask for a picture or an autograph? Yup. Did I mind? Never. I worked hard for them to recognize me, and I was so flattered that they cared about me. That's pretty lucky, and I was thankful for it. That started when I was thirty, and I had turned sixty eight days ago.

And I'd lost a hundred pounds. Today, on my way to the Mississippi, I was stopped exactly once. I was stopped by one guy who wanted to comment on how different I looked and congratulate me on the weight loss—you know, as long as I wasn't sick.

"You're invisible now; you've got no secrets to conceal. How does it feel? How does it feel? To be on your own? Like a complete unknown?" Well, I guess I felt like a rolling stone. I'm typing on a bench on the banks of the Mississippi with a steady stream of people walking by. People who watch TV. They watch *Wizard Wars* and *Fool Us*. They watched *All-Star Celebrity Apprentice*. Some of these people had seen me on TV, but they didn't see me there on the bench.

So, how did it feel? You tell me: how does it feel to walk around a touristy area and watch the people and have them not watch you? How does it feel to get lost in thought and not really think about who you are or who you're supposed to be? I'm the magician who disappeared. I only vanished about a third of my body, but it turns out that's enough to be invisible. Two-thirds of Penn is not critical mass. It's not a quorum. Sixty-six percent of Penn Jillette is not a minyan.

I have great staff. And right now they're working hard. Glenn is already working to book me on TV shows to talk about this book and my weight loss. He'll get me on the cover of magazines holding my big old 44-inch pants around my new skinny waist. He'll make it so that the people walking through the French Quarter stop me again, call me by name, and ask for a picture.

At least I hope we'll be successful. I like being in showbiz. I like people talking to me. I like taking pictures.

But that Friday the thirteenth in New Orleans, I thought: I am invisible now; I have no secrets to conceal.

And it felt pretty fucking good.

Presto! I'm gone.

But I hope I'll be back!

DON'T EXERCISE
(LOSE WEIGHT *AND* FRIENDS)

"There is no god." I've said that sentence on Glenn Beck's TV show in front of his live audience at his studio in the Texas Bible Belt. I've told Republicans that I like immigrants. I've told Democrats that I dig rich people. I've told sane people that I like lawyers.

But nothing I've ever said gets people as crazy as when I say "When you're trying to lose weight, don't exercise." I said that on Dr. Oz's TV show, and he was shocked—and he's hard to shock. My friend Dr. Oz has a really high tolerance for people saying crazy, fucked-up, misleading, wrong shit on his show, but "Don't exercise" really threw him.

It sure is one of CrayRay's most startling rules: "No exercise until you reach your target weight."

Even after reaching your target weight, CrayRay doesn't push for the gym. He doesn't think we should all just sit around, of course—we should take a walk, be active, but we don't really need to go sweat our newly attractive asses off. Americans are accepting the no god and smaller government things slowly but surely, but man, we sure don't want to give up that weight loss is all grunting, sweating, and chewing. We've been told to eat small, high-protein meals really often to "keep your metabolism up" (whatever the fuck that's supposed to mean), and to exercise our asses off. Sweat off those pounds! But sucking "protein" and sweating is body-building, and I was trying to body-downsize.

Those who ridicule complicated weight loss advice always say something along the lines of "Alls you gotta do is eat less and exercise more." That's what we said on our *Bullshit!* show about diet. We were smug about it. And I think it's one of the things we were wrong about. We promised to do a *Penn & Teller: Bullshit of Bullshit!* show as our last show in the series, but we walked away for a better deal and didn't know when we did our last show that it was our last show. We still have hopes of going back and fixing some stuff about climate change, weight loss, secondhand smoke, and other things . . . but I really just want to show a shot of us and say, "And then there are these assholes," in voiceover. Many people wised up before us that you can't outrun your mouth; that you absolutely cannot exercise enough to be able to eat an extra doughnut, but very few of us have taken the next step of saying, "Exercise has nothing to do with weight loss." Weight loss and body-building are two different things that do not work well together.

I know people who want to lose just a few pounds, and they exercise for seven *hours* a week or more, following a cross-training program until the sweat pours off them and spending a shit-ton of money on personal trainers. CrayRay will explain all this in his book (you know, one of those books by a scientist with, you know, like, information and shit in it), but you burn more fat sitting still, or even sleeping, than by exercising hard. You don't burn more calories, but your body burns more fat. We can't stop exercising. I'm not preaching that kind of crazy. Exercise is really good for us. Exercise is necessary for health. We are designed to be active. Our bodies need to work.

But for fat fucks trying to lose weight, exercise can help you hold on to fat as it builds muscles. I spent three months without exercising, and that's when I lost the bulk of my weight. That's the time I spent getting healthy.

This gets into all of CrayRay's stuff about "metabolic winter." In the summer, we run around and eat a lot and store some fat, and then in winter we sit around and use that fat to stay alive. That's what all animals do. But humans have conquered winter. The three big battlefields for all life are dark, cold, and starvation. We've made our whole world light, warm, and full of food. We have won all the battles, and now it's coming back to bite our fat asses. Our bodies live in summer all the time, while we keep preparing for a winter that never comes. It took one single CrayRay "winter" for my body to use up thirty summers' worth of stored fat and get ready to run around again. It was great. When I was on my potato famine, I didn't force myself to exercise. I forced myself to sleep and watch the Stooges. Yup—there was a lack of energy for a while, and CrayRay had me embrace that.

Happily and lazily, I followed CrayRay's convenient advice, and when I hit my target weight, I was really weak. I had lost muscle and strength along with the fat. I couldn't do any push-ups, and even at my fattest I could usually bang out twenty. All my muscles felt so different. I felt like I had to learn to juggle all over again. But once I did a little exercise at my target weight, everything came back so quickly. It took about a month of the *New York Times* seven-minute workout every other day (that's about one hour and forty-five minutes total) for my push-ups to come right back up and my muscles to feel cleaner. They were Iggy Pop muscles and not pro-wrestling muscles, but even I don't know what that means. It took a few hours of juggling for that to come back. I felt strong again in no time. Building muscle and endurance on a thin body is wicked easy.

I've been at my target weight for a year, and I work my arms really intensely—slow-motion reps with weights for about eight minutes every Monday. Yeah; just eight miserable minutes a week. That plus the Monday, Wednesday, and Friday seven-minute workouts puts me at twenty-nine minutes of exercise a week. It's really almost nothing, and I feel great. I should add in a few more walks and maybe a little running, but I'm so happy with how I feel. I try to stay active. When the children want to run around, I run around with them. I take stairs two at a time.

You've finally done it. You found a book that has told you not to exercise. Too bad the book is written by an idiot.

TOUGH GUYS DON'T DANCE

Tough guys don't dance because they're too fucking fat. I believe that gumption, moxie, focus, ambition—you know, toughness—get in the way of health. The very same qualities that can give you a bit of success can also contribute to your being way unhealthy. I bent over backward to name this chapter after the title of a movie I was in so I could write a bit about it; I'll get back to diet in a bit. *Tough Guys Don't Dance* is a weird-ass movie by Norman Mailer. I have no idea if it's good. I have no idea if it's even watchable. I think a few people believe it's pure genius. I don't know about that, but it's crazy, crazy, crazy, and I always love that. Norman Mailer brought me in and said he wrote the part for me. It was a Southern preacher with an enormous cock. I told him I was an atheist from New England. He said, "I'll write the words, you learn the accent, and we'll use a wide-angle lens." I worked so hard on the accent, but I have no idea how much it helped. Some of my Southern friends say I nailed it, some say I didn't. I don't know. I worked with a dialect coach in NYC who had worked with Meryl

Streep. You can see the clip on YouTube. I'm not very good, but I worked hard on it, and that's where it ties in with my eating.

I got to play the husband of Isabella Rossellini. Holy fuck. And I fell in love with Debra Sandlund on the set, but she wasn't fond of me. I got to be in a room with both of them making sex noises on a bed. It was pretty fun. I have a private heartbreaking story about shooting that movie. If we're ever hanging out and I'm in the mood to bum your shit, I'll tell you in person.

Yeah, Isabella Rossellini. If you're ever watching *Blue Velvet*, you might think she's pretty sexy in that movie. In person she's a thousand times sexier and even more beautiful. I met her and immediately wrote a bit in our TV special *Don't Try This at Home* just for her. The bit is called Fire for Two, and the idea was for two people to make out and have symbolic sex but do it all with fire-eating. So we'd kiss, but we'd both be eating fire and the flames would move across our mouths. It's the only time I've ever tried to write a sexy bit, and it included really hard fire-eating. I wrote it so I could be close to Isabella again. I didn't end up ever doing it with her, but I'll get to that part of the story in a few paragraphs, and I'll also try to tie this in to my losing weight, but that'll be even deeper in the chapter.

People sometimes come up to me and kindly say, "I love your work." I am flattered and say thanks, but it always makes me laugh. They don't love my work. They love the results of my work. My real work is stupid, boring, embarrassing, and full of failure. The work is in a hot warehouse with Teller and a few other guys sweating and doing things that don't work. I got this great idea for a fire-eating bit. Actually I got the idea, "Boy, I'd like to make out with Isabella Rossellini; I wonder how I could do that without, you know, being more attractive." This basic idea turned into my taking one of my skills—fire-eating—and figuring out how to do that with two people. Could two people both eat fire and kiss with their mouths on fire? Instead of the standard fire-eating trick where I moved fire from a torch to my mouth and then to another torch, could I add another mouth into that chain? And could that other mouth belong to Isabella Rossellini? That was the idea. That was the bit. Here was the work on that idea: About my best and oldest friend is Robbie Libbon. We've known each other since we both worked at Six Flags Great Adventure amusement park in New Jersey in the '70s. He was doing sword-fighting stunts as one of the Three Musketeers and I was juggling with my partner, Mac-Arthur Genius Grant juggler Michael Moschen. We were all nineteen years old. Robbie and I became good friends, and after he worked with the Big Apple Circus for a few years he came on board with the *Penn & Teller Show*, and we've been working together ever since.

Way back in those Great Adventure Jersey times, Robbie and I decided to learn to eat fire together. Neither of us knew jack shit, but we had a book. We learned fire-eating from a book. This is not a story for National Literacy Month. Books are fine, but don't fucking learn fire-eating from them. It wasn't even a book—it was a fucking pamphlet called *Fire Magic* or something like that. But there's no "magic." There's nothing you can coat your mouth with, there's no "cold fire," no trick torches. Fire-eating is just a stupid skill. And if you want to learn this skill from a book, you better be a couple of teenagers willing to burn the shit out of yourselves. The book didn't explain how to make the torches, so we tried tying cotton onto metal rods with nylon thread. Nylon that melted, stuck to our mouths and lips, and burned until it hardened, and then burned us longer. The burning nylon left marks. So we switched from nylon to wire and turned our torches into branding irons. That left marks and blisters. But we were tough guys, and we kept going. At the end of this Robbie/Penn adventure, we were really shitty fire-eaters with mouths that looked very damaged and diseased. My girlfriend at the time was also nineteen years old and up for anything sexually—we were freaks—but even she wouldn't kiss me for a few days. Yecch. It wasn't until a real carny, my buddy Doc Swan, taught me real-world fire-eating that my mouth didn't have oozing blisters every time I tried it. Doc also taught me tricks that looked good. Books suck.

Sometime during Robbie's Big Apple days he also learned fire-eating the right way. If you see the movie *Annie* (and why would you?) he's the fire-eater in the big scene that also has Michael Moschen juggling in it. Even doing it right, Robbie burned the living shit out of himself that day. He's a pro. One can get good at fire-eating, but it's never a smart thing to do.

I did not get the idea for the two-person fire-eating routine so I could make out with Robbie Libbon. I got the idea for Fire for Two so I could make out with Isabella Rossellini. But I had to make sure that the fire-eating mouth transfer would work. Robbie Libbon and I engaged in another fire-eating adventure. This time we didn't have a book. We were inventing tricks that even Doc Swan didn't know. Our work that week was to sit on a hard bench together—two old friends in a sweaty warehouse, again in Jersey ("A Great State To Do Stupid Shit" should be their motto)—burning the shit out of each other. We sat for hours making it clear to each other that the making out was fake and the pain was real. Showbiz is awkward and painful. The idea for two-person fire-eating was beautiful in my head, and the goal of making out with Isabella Rossellini was noble, but the path was neither. Robbie and I sat side by side with our arms around each other, singeing each other's eyebrows and nose hair off. We would breathe in the stench of each other's burning flesh and nose hairs mixed with each other's petroleum burps. It smelled disgusting. It looked disgusting, too, as we had to watch blisters develop on each other's lips and ooze to the point where a horny girlfriend wouldn't even talk to us. We did our flaming kisses over and over until we figured it out. Sickening. It also hurt like holy hell at the time and for days after. I'm telling you, Isabella is that attractive, and we're tough guys.

When Robbie and I had learned the tricks and felt we could teach them to a beginner, I got Isabella's phone number from her agent and gave her a call. I explained the gag and told her very honestly and in great detail that even if she were taught well and carefully, even if she did everything right, she would still get burned. Her professionally beautiful lips—the most beautiful lips in the world—would be burned. The lips that Revlon paid more to photograph than they'd ever paid before would be blistered if she worked on this bit with me. She said, "I'd love to do that with you." And you thought she couldn't be sexier! Our agents started setting up the deal for her to be in our NBC special later that year, and we started planning a time for her to watch Robbie and me do the bit and learn to do it so her beautiful lips would have time to heal. Find something beautiful and hurt it—that's the way I live.

Because there's no god and we live in a random universe full of pain, I never ended up doing the bit with Isabella. She got a part in a big fancy-schmancy movie that was shooting in Russia while we were shooting our little TV special in NYC . . . and I think Revlon also didn't want their zillion-dollar lips burned by carny trash. Really hard to blame them. When Isabella called me to tell me she couldn't do it, she also told me that if I did it with anyone else, she would consider it cheating and never forgive me. We had already promised it to NBC, though, so I had to do it without Isabella. The bad news is that Isabella and I have never really hung out since. I don't believe she holds me not burning her against me; our paths just haven't crossed. The good news is that we ended up doing the bit with a Victoria's Secret model who is also beautiful beyond belief and was my girlfriend. Beautiful beyond belief, with beautiful lips, and we burned the shit out of her. The bad news is we broke up. But the best news is I ended up with EZ, my wife, and when we do the bit now, EZ has me do it with Georgie, our Vegas show-woman who does a lot of bits with us in the *Penn & Teller Show.* My wife's lips stay perfect. Georgie and I are pretty good at fire-eating by now and we don't get burned that much, but we still get tagged every few shows. My mouth and lips get burned, and I don't give a fuck because I'm a tough guy.

The conventional wisdom is that it takes a tough guy to diet and exercise. It takes willpower to decide to take control of one's body and be healthy, but that's not the way it seems to me. When I was obese, everything was hard—everything—and I can handle hard. It was hard to do the show, but that's okay. It was hard to play with my children, but I still did. It was hard to fucking breathe, but I kept breathing. If I were a wimp, I wouldn't have put up with that shit. If I weren't tough, I would have gone to the doctor and said, "I can't go through every single fucking day with every single fucking breath being hard. My children are energetic, and I play with them and it kills me. I do a two-hour show every night and I'm panting just doing the monologues. Getting up in the morning is a fucking chore. What do I need to do to fix this?" The doc would have said I had to stop eating like a pig, and things would be easier. But I could handle tough. I got through. My parents taught me that my job matters and I have to do it no matter what. I've done irresponsible shows with fevers of way over a hundred degrees. I've left the stage to vomit in a bucket and come back on and continued without the audience being any wiser. I've had a full EKG hookup on me and O_2 tanks and masks and paramedics backstage to get me through shows. I've gotten dressed for the show while shaking so badly that I needed help to stand up. I've done the show with broken bones and with my hand burned so badly I needed a glove taped over it so the skin wouldn't peel off onstage. I did the show the night my father died. I did the show the night my mother died. I did the show the night my sister died. I toughed through the death show trifecta. I'm a tough motherfucker. I've never hit anyone in anger, but I can take a punch. I've blown my voice out and had steroid shots just to be able to get a single tone out, and did the whole show in that monotone and still got laughs. I've done the show hating Teller and with Teller justifiably hating me, and we worked together. I've done the show when the tricks weren't working and the crowd had had enough of me, and I didn't stop. I sure as fuck could do the show forever no matter how fat I was. If I hadn't been so tough, my fat would have gotten in the way of the show and I would have fixed it. Someone would have made me fix it. There are livelihoods riding on that show.

My family matters to me. If my fat had gotten in the way of playing with my children, I would have fixed it. But I'm tough enough that even being fat and feeling like shit, I could pick up my children and run around. My heart would pound, my head would throb, and I would pant, but I would not not play with my children. I owed them a dad who played with them, and I was tough enough to deliver that, even as fat as I was. If I had felt that being fat got in the way of me being their dad, I would have fixed it.

I was lying to myself, of course. The truth is that being fat fucked me up in every way possible. It made me less good as a performer and as a dad. It fucked me up as a husband, as a coworker, and as a human being. When I lost the hundred pounds, everything got easier and better. I lost the weight and found a kind of happiness I had forgotten I could feel. Each of my children weighs less than a hundred pounds. At the instant I hit my target weight, both of my children together weighed just a little more than I had lost. I could hold both of my children together in my arms and run with the same effort it used to take to just move my own solitary fat ass. Without that hundred-plus pounds, I smiled bigger, more sincerely, and more often, with less effort. I was easier to get along with. I was funnier. I was kinder.

Everything was easier when I was happier, and I was happier when everything was easier. But the tough guy had thought that as long as I was getting through, I was okay. I thought that things worth doing, like having a family and a career, weren't supposed to be easy. I didn't care how hard they were, I was going to do them.

It wasn't that I didn't know being fat was hard. It wasn't that I thought losing weight was going to be hard work. One of the problems was that I was tough enough to get through no matter what, at least until my fucking heart stopped dead and/or I stroked out. As long as I was conscious, I would do the show and be a dad.

Now that I think back on it, I kind of *felt*—I could never *think* this, it's too stupid—that taking care of myself was the easy way out. I felt that respecting my body and my energy would make me a loser. Only wimps paid attention to their health and were careful about what they ate. Assholes would have to ask the waiter at the restaurant for steamed vegetables with nothing on them. Tough guys would say, "I don't care; bring me any food you have lying around," and then eat it. I never sent anything back to any kitchen. I didn't care. I wasn't so weak that I had to have a salad waiting for me after our show; I'd just get a room-service cheeseburger and some fries and hit the hay. That's what a tough guy did. And when I got the blood pressure dial tones in my head and could feel the silent killer yelling in my ears? Fuck it. I got up and did my work. Strap 110 pounds around my waist and I'll still get through my day and do my tasks. I could do the *Penn & Teller Show* with a dozen lead baseball bats shoved way up my fat ass.

All I had to do to lose that weight was convince myself that losing the weight was not the easy way out but the hard way out. I had to convince myself that it took a tough guy to take care of himself. That's what CrayRay gave me. He didn't say, "Hey, dieting is easy and fun." He made it clear to me that what I was going to do would be tough and crazy. I would eat only potatoes. I would cut my calories to almost nothing. I would feel hungry a lot. I would have to fight my old habits every second of every day. He made it clear that most people failed at what I was going to do. He made it clear that losing weight was more difficult than dragging my fat ass around for the rest of my shorter life.

All I needed to do to be able to channel my personality into losing the weight was to simply believe that losing the weight would take more willpower than living my life as an obese fuck.

Tough guys can dance. Tough guys get healthy.

HIGHER THAN A KITE AND SICKER THAN A DOG: NOT GENETICS—JUST A FAT FUCK

Every couple of years P&T play Lake Tahoe. It's over a mile up—6,224 feet above sea level. It's a nice room and nice audiences, but I would always get altitude sickness. I would get it bad. From the first few hours after arriving, I'd have headaches and couldn't walk up stairs without stopping to rest. I was weak and miserable the whole time. I once flew directly from Tahoe to L.A. on a smoggy day and was so thrilled to be able to feel the air going into my lungs. I hated the altitude.

Many years ago, on one of our gigs there, my altitude sickness must have coupled with a virus or something. Before the show, I was backstage having what felt like a fucking seizure. I was shaking so violently I couldn't get dressed. Jeff Ross, who opened for us that night, was onstage killing. Soon he would throw it to us, and I'd have to do the show. But I couldn't stand up. I was sweating and burning up and freezing. I'm telling you, it was tied to the altitude. Every time I was in a high-altitude city, I felt like shit the whole time—not this bad, but I'm sure whatever it was this time was started by being on top of fucking Everest.

Casinos used to be run by criminals. Back then, I would have had a guy with a broken nose backstage saying, "Listen, asshole, toughen the fuck up. It's a full house out there, and we do not give money back. Put your clothes on and get your ass out onstage, magic boy! It's showtime."

Now corporations run casinos. To my buddies who feel the Bern, these are the same, but to me there is a difference. In the corporate casino world, there's more paperwork. When I couldn't stop myself from shaking, Teller called an ambulance, and two EMTs arrived, glued EKG disks to my chest, and got me on a gurney. Just a few seconds after they entered, as I was being strapped in, another guy arrived. He was a nice guy with a tie and a smile and an unbroken nose. He had a piece of paper with him, which he read to me. I don't remember exactly what he said, but what he read made a difference. This was something that had been written by lawyers and then vetted by other lawyers and bounced off another set of lawyers and probably tested in a court of civil law. The nice guy with the tie read that the casino's primary concern was my health. That was all that mattered. Not only did they not want me to do a show if it would threaten my health, but they would furthermore not *allow* me to do a show that would put my health in any jeopardy. They were ready, willing, and able (and desirous) to have Jeff make an announcement that I was sick, and they would refund every penny. The EMTs said, "Great, let's get him to the hospital."

But the nice guy with the tie had more explaining to do. It was, *of course*, my decision. It was a sold-out crowd, and they were really excited for a P&T magic show (I think he was ad-libbing off some boilerplate). The EMTs tried to point out that the decision had been made and I was going into the ambulance. The nice guy with the tie continued to explain that I still had my rights, and there was a big crowd and after all I was in showbiz and maybe I wanted to have the show go on.

I told the EMTs that I might want to give it a try, and they began reciting their own boilerplate. They had been called for an emergency. They had examined me, and I was wicked fucked-up (I don't remember the exact wording), and in their opinion I needed to take their ambulance to the hospital. Nice guy with the tie said as long as I was conscious, it was my choice. The EMTs said that once they had been called, they could not be dismissed by anyone other than me. I told everyone in the room the deal: if I could stand up long enough to get dressed, I would go on. The nice guy with the tie said, "That is entirely your personal choice; you are, of course, assuming all responsibility and culpability yourself, and I'm going to need you to sign this little piece of paper saying the casino, all its owners, employees, shareholders, hookers, mascots, and pets have advised you to cancel the show," or something like that. I stood up, and the EMTs made me sign something that said they had been falsely called and that nothing was wrong with me. I affirmed that I was in good health. They all then helped me to stand up and held me while I got dressed.

The nice guy with the tie told the EMTs to stay for the show and keep the ambulance right outside the stage door. He told them to give me oxygen whenever I was offstage and to keep the EKG discs on me and check me while I huffed O_2 during Teller's solo bits. That's what happened. I don't remember the show, but I guess I made it through. Jeff Ross still thanks me for letting him do a few extra minutes. I was dying; he was killing. Right after the show, the EMTs and my buddy Robbie got me into an ambulance and I was taken to the hospital, where everyone waited for me to have a heart attack. I didn't, but I felt awful. It was a bad night for everyone.

No other trip up high was as dramatic as that one, but when I was at the Sundance Film Festival in Park City, Utah, with my movie *The Aristocrats*, I was seven thousand feet up and landed in the hospital. My partners Provenz and Pete Golden hurried over to let me know that my health came first, but we *had* spent a lot of money to set up those press hits. When I took our movie *Tim's Vermeer* to Telluride (what the fuck is it with film festivals being so high up?), I was up 8,700 feet and felt like shit, and that was after I had taken the drug Diamox for a few days to try to ward off the altitude sickness.

Of course, I thought my problem with altitude sickness was genetic, like all the rest of my fat-fuck problems. I was just unlucky to not be able to function high up. It was something to do with my fucking Newfoundland blood or something. I never admitted that I was simply a fat fuck. When Sam Kinison played Tahoe he needed oxygen backstage, and wasn't he a fat fuck, too? I guess I should have learned from that, but I was also told that Tiffany used oxygen backstage when she was seventeen years old and weighed as much as my left leg and sang her just-faster-enough-to-not-be-sexy version of "I Think We're Alone Now." I told myself it wasn't weight; it was just the luck of the draw. Man, I told myself that about everything. Such a self-deluding asshole.

I weighed 229 pounds when my movie *Director's Cut* (you know, the one I had gained the 110 pounds for) opened Slamdance. That festival is also in Park City, so also seven thousand feet up. EZ and the long-suffering Glenn both reminded me to take Diamox for a couple of days before we left, but I said fuck it. I didn't want to bother; but also a part of me knew all along that my high-altitude problem was really a fat-fuck problem. I didn't take any Diamox.

I flew to Park City and we premiered our movie. I did interviews and pictures up and down the main street and trotted up flights of stairs next to the perfectly fit and always handsome Harry Hamlin. Neither of us was puffing. No huffing O_2. No EKG discs. No headaches. No seizures. No EMTs or nice guys with ties reading from scripts or buddies telling me all they cared about was my health, but shouldn't I just do what I promised I would do. There was no problem.

I guess someone could have screamed in my face that I was a fat fuck and that being a fat fuck would kill me even faster on top of a mountain than at sea level. But no one did. There was no nice guy with a tie saying that one of my primary concerns should be my own health, because the casino, all its owners, employees, shareholders, my family, friends, hookers, mascots, and pets had to take care of their own fucking lives, and who the fuck was I to make all these people waste their time taking care of a fat fuck on a mountain?

FUHRBURGER

Unlike CrayRay, Dr. Joel Fuhrman is a real, no-kidding medical Doctor Doctor Mister MD. He also came in third place at the World Professional Pairs Figure Skating Championship in Spain in 1976, skating with his sister. I don't have a joke about that, but I don't need one; it's just funny.

Joel is called "Fuhrburger" by no one other than me, and even I don't call him that to his face, but this is my fucking book, so fuck him, he's Fuhrburger. Fuhrburger may be more than bug-nutty. He might be kinda sorta an alternative medicine whack job, but I really like him. His diet is pretty much all I eat now. It's possible that if I were still doing *Penn & Teller: Bullshit!*, I would introduce him with "Then there's *this* asshole" and rip him a new one. That was my job then, and Fuhrburger does stuff that we could have crushed him with. He seems to believe that everything can be cured with the right magic food, and he's even said some dangerous, weird-ass shit about the flu vaccine, and I'm afraid to dig too deeply into what he's said about other vaccines. Howard Stern once told me he couldn't get to know anyone, because he'd end up liking them and not be able to do his job. Maybe that happened with Stern and Trump, but I don't follow either of them closely enough.

I've spent a couple of hours with Fuhrburger and I really like him, and I think he's right about a lot of stuff. *Bullshit!* is no longer my job, so I can be nuanced. That doesn't mean I don't call bullshit. I still try to be as honest as I can. When I had Fuhrburger on *Penn's Sunday School,* I busted him on some of his crazier cancer claims and his blaming of everything on diet, but on *P&T: BS!* I wouldn't have just busted some things he said, I would have taken all of him down. Let's say we "rounded up" on the bullshit. If someone was 65 percent full of shit, we'd call them totally full of shit for comedic purposes (and it was a half-hour show). In my real life I tend to round the good parts of people up. If someone has a couple of ideas that I like among lots of shit, I try to focus on the good ideas. It seems healthier, but not as funny. When I'm not on TV I go back to embracing my love of people on the fringes. And I'm not even sure that Fuhrburger is that far on the fringes anymore. The sensible, empirical science-diet epicenter may be moving over to where Fuhrburger has been hanging for years. That doesn't mean he's right, but he sure is wicked thin and very healthy, and you're better off taking diet advice from a thin, healthy fuck than from a fat fuck.

CrayRay grabbed me by the potato balls and dragged me down to my target weight, but since getting there, I pretty much eat Fuhrburger. EZ and I have all his books and are premium members of his website (we paid! But even if we hadn't, I'd still call him "bug-nutty," even though it's an animal product when I bite the hand that feeds me). We get new recipes every day, and EZ tries a lot of them and we come back to some of them over and over. We eat his dill pea soup every week. It's my comfort food, the new grilled cheese for me. His recipes sometimes cheat a little by CrayRay's philosophy, but they mostly stay whole plants: no animal products, no refined grains, stupid-low salt, oil, and sugar. Fuhrburger likes his food bland. He likes the flavors in the plants. His idea of spicy is a little rosemary or something. So we load in the cayenne and Tabasco and rock that way. But a lot of the stuff is great right off the page, now that we've lost our SOS (Salt, Oil, Sugar) habituation.

He has recipes with names like "Doctor Fuhrman's Famous Anti-Cancer Soup," and he has special potions for immunity. He'll tell you that the SAD diet is full of cooties and his diet fights those cooties. Yeah, he puts it in fancy scientific terms, but he means "cooties." The nuts who study "blue zones," where people live the longest, say those old cats and kitties eat mostly vegetarian with lots and lots of beans, and that's Fuhrburger. Folks in the blue zones who live longer than the rest of us also put family first, and I'm down with that; purpose in life really matters, and I have that in spades. Physical work and religion are also important, and . . . um . . . let's get back to Fuhrburger. So, I don't know about all of Fuhrburger's potions and elixirs. I know that anecdotal evidence means jack shit, but I just don't get sick much anymore. I take hay fever pills a couple of times a year instead of every day for months; my arthritis is way, way better; and I've gotten just one very light cold since I've been on his food—and I used to get a bad one almost every month. But the honest answer is, I don't know. I'm keeping the weight off, and with some spice we really like his food, so we do it.

Some of my skeptic buddies have busted Fuhrburger for being on Dr. Oz's insane TV show. Well, I've been on Dr. Oz's insane TV show, and I'll go on again to talk about using Withings products, and if he invites me, I'll go on again to pimp this book. When I was still in high school I saw Jean Shepherd speak at a college in Amherst, Massachusetts. I used to skip high school and drive to the local college and sit in on classes to see guest speakers. Jean was a hero of mine, the greatest storyteller on radio. He's now mostly known as the guy who wrote and narrated *A Christmas Story*. It's a fine movie, but I like his trippier radio stuff more. The radio reception up in Greenfield for his NYC show was so weak I had to hold my radio antenna just right and cozy up to his perfect voice with my little radio speaker against my ear. After his talk at UMass he had a Q&A, and someone called him out for having his stories published in the sexist magazine, *Playboy*. Jean didn't address the morality of *Playboy* at all. He said that sometimes when he uses a urinal there's stuff written on the wall above it that he doesn't agree with, but he still uses it. That's one argument. A hero of mine, Tommy Smothers, busted me for going on Glenn Beck's show. He said that if Hitler had a talk show, I would have gone on it. I said, "Yes, I would have told the truth." I don't agree with Glenn Beck and I go on his show, and I've said on that show "There is no god." I don't agree with Bill Maher on vaccines and other stuff, but I've gone on his shows a lot. I costarred on *The Celebrity Apprentice* for two seasons with Trump . . . but that was before I heard his campaign speeches and read his hateful tweets. Maybe I'd have to draw the line below Hitler but above Trump. Although if he asks me to be on his post-losing-presidential-run show, I'll probably go on; what do I care?

When I ate hamburgers, In-N-Out Burger had Christian shit right on their cups, and was I sure I agreed with everything the owners of White Castle believed? A lot of good Christians (I mean "good" not to intensify "Christian" but to contrast with it) come to our show and they know we're atheists; but they still want to see our magic show.

I'm aware all of this is very facile and convenient. By going on Dr. Oz and Glenn Beck, I give my insignificant imprimatur to their shows. But I also give my point of view to their audiences as honestly as I can. If I were president of the United States of America (and I would be better than Trump, but worse than Hitler), I would have to think more about what it means for me to go on those shows, but at my level of sub-star, I go where I'm booked. I think I can give Fuhr-burger the same pass.

I know Fuhrburger doesn't agree with me on everything, but here he is in my book. And we both disagree with Dr. Oz, but we both go on his show. I'm sure Fuhrburger is wrong about a lot, because food is complicated, but I love his books and his recipes. It would be wrong for me to not give him credit for the help he's given me with my diet.

And I like him and love that he figure-skated with his sister.

UNETHICAL VEGAN? PLANT HOLE?

I don't really have a good name for how I eat. I don't eat any animal products (except "Rare and Appropriate"), so I am, by definition, "vegan." Except I'm not a vegan. The idea is not not to eat animals; the idea is to eat healthy. Not eating animals isn't the impetus, it's a side effect. Calling myself a vegan would be like calling myself a cultural Christian. Yes, I'm an American, I went to church as a child, and I happen to follow much of the morality of modern Christianity—not because it's Christian, but because modern Christianity mostly follows natural and logical human morality. If you look at how American Christians dress and speak and act in daily life, I follow all that. I have the same problem with the label "Cultural Jew." People use that term to mean that they were brought up Jewish and that the food and the culture and the history are still important to them even if they're not practicing the religion. The idea is that somehow loving one's family and liking Lenny Bruce and peppering one's speech with American Yiddish is what makes one Jewish.

So if I love my family and like *Stroker Ace* and pepper my speech with "Hey, buddy, fuck all y'all," I'm a cultural Christian? No. Being Christian or Jewish is not a race or a culture, it's a religion. The cultural part of being a Jew I've happily adopted. I claim Lenny Bruce and Bob Dylan as part of my culture. I also add in Sun Ra and Jimi Hendrix even though I don't identify culturally as African American. I also claim Salman Rushdie even though I wasn't raised Muslim and Ayaan Hirsi Ali and Richard Dawkins even though I wasn't born and raised in Africa. Saul Bellow asked (off the cuff, and he didn't really stand by it), "Who is the Tolstoy of the Zulus?" Ralph Wiley answered, "Tolstoy is the Tolstoy of the Zulus," and ended that jive-ass tribalism with one perfect sentence.

Growing up with Brylcreem and *Cannonball Run* doesn't make me a cultural Christian, and not eating animal products doesn't make me vegan. If one doesn't actively believe in god, one is not a Christian or a Jew of any kind. And if one doesn't think it's morally wrong to use animals for food or clothing, one is not vegan. Vegan restaurants are harder for me to eat at than steak houses. Vegan restaurants seem to love the SOS. Some vegan restaurants try to duplicate shitty food without using animal products. To a fellow like me, that's the same as serving Big Macs and fries. Steak houses can get me some plain vegetables and one of my beloved potatoes, and we're done. In the good *The Producers* (the original movie with Gene Wilder), to show how poor he is, Zero Mostel screams, "I'm wearing a cardboard belt!" When people ask if I'm a vegan, I try to answer, in the same tone, "I'm wearing a leather belt!"

Fuhrburger calls the way I eat "nutritarian," and that's like trying to call Sixth Avenue "Avenue of the Americas"—it just ain't going to catch on. "CroNut," coined after CrayRay's last name, Cronise, is just an in-joke. Someone suggested "evidence-based diet," and unless that someone has the muscle it takes to push "black" to "African American," that's not going to happen, either.

I self-identify as atheist, but it's really a shitty label because it doesn't get its definition from anything positive. As they say, how can not collecting stamps be a hobby? We had the term "Dead Head" for people who loved the Grateful Dead, but we don't define those of us who love Dylan, Stravinsky, and Sun Ra as Non–Dead Heads. The positive way to state my diet philosophy is "I eat whole plants." "WholePlanter"? "Plant-Whole"? I kind of like that. "I'm a plant-whole"; maybe I'll try that, but I don't think it really swings.

Mac King, Goudeau, and Andy really like "unethical vegan." They like that it abbreviates to "UV." That's nice, but it's not really right. There are some ethical benefits to being a plant-hole (yeah, I don't like that, either). I drive a Leaf, an all-electric car. Teller drives a Tesla; he's the fancy guy without a family to support. I don't feel like I'm saving the earth by doing it. I know that an electric car doesn't mean "zero emissions," it means no tailpipe emissions. But still, the power comes from somewhere, and that somewhere is most likely spewing carbon into the air. If stupid hippies hadn't killed nuclear power, we'd have nuclear power plants, safer and cheaper than coal-fired plants, all over, and electric cars really would be zero emissions. You want to blame carbon emissions on someone, blame them on Bruce Springsteen and the Clash—they did that rocking "No Nukes" concert. We need hippie tie-dyed nuclear power plants and everyone driving electric cars. I drive an electric car because they're quiet and I hate gas stations. I like plugging my car in at home, and I fucking *love* plugging my car in at work. The Rio All-Suites Hotel and Casino has a charging station just for me, and they don't bill me for the energy. So, when I plug in, I'm sticking it to the man! I drive an electric car because Obama put in one of his many incentives that just give money to the well-off.

I shouldn't get tax breaks more than anyone else, but Obama's tax breaks for electric cars benefit only people wealthy enough to have a second car. I can have an electric car only because my wife has a gasoline-powered car that'll go far enough for us to not have to plan our whole day around staying within sixty miles of home. Teller has a second car *and* his Tesla goes over two hundred miles on a charge. Teller needs a tax break less than I do. We don't need the tax breaks, but we take them and figure it's a few bucks less that our government can use to kill people in our name.

Electric cars don't save the environment as much as they should (because of the Boss), but having mine does help an itty-bitty teensy-weensy bit. I don't think it's morally wrong to use animals for food, but the animal suffering that happens at factory farms sure is bothersome. I don't think animal suffering is even measured on the same moral scale as human suffering, but it's still suffering, and it hurts my heart. I don't even have to go to morality (although that argument may very well be valid); I can just go to aesthetics. Factory farming is really not pleasing to look at or even to think about. My children still eat meat (we're working on them), but I like that my tiny little footprint got a little smaller with my new diet.

We did a *Bullshit!* episode over ten years ago in which we shrugged at climate change. Because of that, every time one of our scientist buddies says something nice about us, there are two people who post something like "Penn & Teller rolled their collective eyes many years ago at climate change and must be shunned in perpetuity. Don't let them change their minds!" on Twitter. (I know that's 143 characters; I guess they don't use the words "collective" or "perpetuity.") The truth is that Penn & Teller were never climate change deniers. We just didn't know. Since then, peer pressure and kowtowing to authority have shut us the fuck up. We drive electric cars. I can also try to placate the climate people by calling myself a vegan. Eating onions imported from

Mexico leaves a smaller carbon footprint than eating local chickens. As we keep working on our children's diets and on growing our little vegetable garden, the Jillettes will very soon be giving the polar bears room to play badminton with their icy sub-zero shuttlecocks on massive ice floes.

AND, OH YEAH, BY THE WAY—MY HAIR FELL OUT

Okay, I'm off a lot of blood pressure meds, I sleep better, I have more energy, I can play with my children, my eczema is better, my arthritis is better, and I'm happier, but . . . my fucking hair fell out.

I've always had great hair. Even when I was a fat fuck, people dug my hair. Men, women, and children would ask to run their hands through my hair. The color wasn't real—I dyed it so it was kind of Wayne Newton black—but it really grew out of my head. I was in my late fifties, and my hairline ran right straight across the front of my forehead. After a day in the wind, you couldn't get a comb through it. My hair was thick, plentiful, and long—hanging down my back, curling on my shoulders. I was able to bang ten inches to "Locks of Love" and still have enough hanging to be sexy.

Well, I lost a hundred pounds, and all of a sudden I could get a comb through my hair. It was getting easier to comb and brush. Maybe losing a hundred pounds had made me stronger. Hair and makeup took less time, and the big old squirrel tail hanging down my back was more subdued. My manager, Glenn, was the first to tell me I was losing my fucking hair.

I was in denial. I told him no way.

I asked my wife.

"Yup, you've lost a lot of your hair."

I asked my hairdresser.

"Yup, you lost a lot of hair when you started losing weight."

I asked our hair and makeup person.

"Yeah, it's a lot thinner."

I was losing my hair.

So I asked CrayRay, "Am I losing my fucking hair?"

"Yeah, you lose a lot of hair with rapid weight loss."

He hadn't billboarded that to me. He was pretty casual about it. He said it would come back after I hit my target weight and increased my calories, that it was just something that happens on extreme low-calorie diets. I'm not sure my hair will come back. I'm not sure all my hair loss is just due to the extreme low-calorie diet. It might also be the invisible hairy hand making an age-market correction. I had been on Minoxidil for my blood pressure, which is the same drug that's used to fight hair loss. I was on a massive dose—75mg every morning, and the same at night. I'd been taking 150mg a day. There isn't much information on what oral—as opposed to topical—Minoxidil does for hair, but I was on it for years. I didn't notice the hair loss from the low-calorie diet at all, really, but others noticed it after I was off the Minoxidil. So, I don't know. I just don't know.

Now that I'm eating a shit-ton of calories, maybe my hair will come back. But it's not likely I'll go back on Minoxidil, so it might not come back. I'm okay with that, but that's my personality. I tend to accept things pretty quickly. I know a lot of men freak out when their hair starts going away. My dad had hair right up until he died at almost ninety, but it did thin out. I think I like my hair being thinner.

It's easier to brush and comb, and I think it looks okay. I went from a squirrel tail in the back to wearing my hair in a man-bun like some sort of aging Brooklyn hipster. I used to wear my hair down for the pre-show while I played bass and after the show while taking pictures, but now I just keep it up.

It's part of my new look. My new look is recently divorced English professor. I think that's what I'm going for, and man-bun with thinning hair always tied back seems better.

But I'm trying to tell the truth in this book, at least unless it gets in the way of the story, so I had to say that either the diet or coming off the Minoxidil certainly made my hair thinner.

So, now you know that.

SO, WHAT THE FUNK *DO* YOU EAT?

Whole Plants. And funk.

CrayRay, Fuhrburger, and now I have written whole books about what Dr. Michael Klaper prescribes in two words: "Whole plants." Occam's diet book. The "Jesus wept" of diet advice. The Klap can add one verb and another two words and cover all health advice with five words in two sentences: "Eat whole plants. Take walks."

The "whole" part of "whole plants" means not refined. You don't want to throw away any part of the plant that's edible. So, sugar, but with all the fruit around it, and all the water and the fiber, too. Rice, but not just the white part, also the brown and black part. You gotta eat the whole apple, but you don't have to eat the whole tree—that's not edible.

I had to have the "whole plants" part of "whole plants" explained to me, so here's a list of things that aren't whole plants:

ANIMAL PRODUCTS.

"Wait, so what about cheese and eggs?"

"Cheese and eggs are fine as long as you pick them yourself fresh off an organic dairy tree, you fucking idiot."

No Big Macs, no steaks, no veal, no chicken, no chicken fingers, no clams, no salmon, no horsemeat, no tripe, no haggis, no sausage, no lard, no schmaltz, no liver, no Camembert, no Roquefort, no anything in the *Monty Python* Cheese Shop sketch, no Spam, no eggs over easy or sunny-side up or poached or coddled, no quail or ostrich eggs, no honey (a bee is an animal, you moron), and . . . oh dear, no bacon. There is only one exception to this: cum, because god is kind.

REFINED ANYTHING.

"What about pasta and flour?"

"Hey, fuckwad, maybe you have a spaghetti tree in your Brie orchard."

Nope. No angel hair, no elbow macaroni, no fettuccine, no pappardelle, no rotelle, no white rice, no bread, no cupcakes, and, damn, no doughnuts. It's not the "plant" part, it's the "whole" part that takes pasta and cake off the list. But cum is still okay.

SALT.

Salt is a fucking rock, not a plant, knucklehead, but I get lots of it from plants, just not added to plants. Once I was off the jive-ass Standard American Diet, plain celery tasted salty to me. But no added salt, not even in cooking. Again, cum is fine.

OIL.

No frying or sautéing. Oil is not a whole plant; grease is squeezed out of the whole plant or animal and the rest is thrown away or added to hog asshole leftovers and put into the scrapple that Teller fries up for breakfast as a rare treat. So, no vegetable oil, no olive oil, no canola oil, no flax oil, no lard, no coconut oil, no oil oil. I don't use oil for cooking (I don't cook); vegetables are sautéed for me in water or unsalted vegetable broth. I can use a very, very small amount of oil for flavor, but none for cooking. When I say "very, very small amount," I mean about a teaspoon a day, just for flavor. All the weight I lost was on less than a teaspoon of good healthy vegetable oil per hour; just that little bit of oil, no matter how virgin and organic, adds up to about 0.9 pounds a day. It adds up fast, and does a body no good. Lube during sex is fine, but just for flavor; I try to spit out quantities greater than a teaspoon.

SUGAR.

"What about maple syrup?"

Oh dear. This is a tough one for me. I'm from Massachusetts, and regardless of what those liars in Vermont will tell you, Massachusetts has the best maple syrup (and, I guess, now the best heroin). I'm flying my children to New England this spring for sugar on snow at a buddy's maple farm. Sugar on snow is maple syrup taken while it's being refined (that word alone shows you I can't really eat it) and poured onto snow, where it congeals into a wonderful diabetic coma of maple taffy. It's so sweet that it has to be served with Saltines and dill pickles just to cut it a bit (like the baby laxative in heroin—we New Englanders know this shit). I grew up with maple syrup on everything. We were proud of our maple syrup. When I was living in San Francisco in the '80s, my avant-garde music friends from Louisiana would get big bags of pecans from their parents for solstice, while I got a gallon of good Massachusetts maple syrup (which would last me almost the year). You put those Louisiana and Massachusetts treats together, and you've got some fine breakfast pancakes. I will use a "Rare and Appropriate" for sugar on snow when I take my children back East, but maple syrup is not part of my normal diet. No maple products, unless I'm going to eat the whole maple tree. I guess I could drink the sap before it's boiled down; that's kinda just tree water, but it ain't syrup.

So, no maple syrup, no white sugar, no confectioner's sugar, no powdered sugar, no brown sugar, no raw sugar, no agave, no molasses, no stevia. But "whole plants" does include fruit, and fruit, now that I'm off SAD, is really sweet. I can eat a whole fresh watermelon. I love oranges. My favorite meal now is four or five containers of blueberries and blackberries. I rinse them off and throw them into a huge metal bowl, shake on a lot of cayenne pepper and a shit-ton of plain cocoa, and it's like a flourless chocolate cake with berries. Now that I read this, I guess that cayenne and cocoa aren't whole plants . . . um . . . but spices seem okay. It's delicious. I put on enough cayenne that no one but me can eat it. I consider it child repellent. Fruit is the way to feed my sweet tooth—but no dried fruit. Raisins, apricots, prunes, dried pears, dried anything are not whole plants; they're missing water, and I need that to fill me up. And no fruit juices at all, because that's too much water . . . and no fruit . . . and lots of sugar. No dried fruit or wet fruit; I guess that's what I mean. Just fruit.

Whole plants, CrayRay, and my doctor got me really healthy. I was a new Penn. Healthy, trim, energetic, happy Penn. I had no cravings. I fought the advertising and the social pressure to be constantly fed. Dr. Fuhrburger's recipes all have this clean, healthful feel. I like feeling clean and healthy. I like my stomach working right and my skin clearing up and my arthritis going away. I love the health.

But I missed the funk.

Animal products are funky. Whether you're talking about a rare steak or a piece of wicked smelly cheese, there is something not quite right about eating animal products, and that's the best part of eating them. Eating meat and cheese is like good fucking. Even if you are totally sex positive and embrace your inner slut and do no shaming and are happy to add a few more letters to your LGBT sandwich, you still want sex to be dirty. Sex needs to bring da funk. It needs to have looks, smells, feels, tastes, and sounds that have a top note of disgusting. Anal sex and blue cheese are for grown-ups. There's a kind of jaded, world-weary, something-not-quite-right vibe to the best kinds of sex. You can fuck right after a shower and in the daylight by a clear mountain stream with a blindfolded string quartet playing live, and it should still be dirty. You can't have great sex without the funk. Not just sex—you don't want any music without funk. Auto-tune and beat grids have to be used judiciously. We want a little tension on the beat and a little wobble in the intonation. Dirty reminds us we're alive. It reminds us that we're animals, and animals are funky. They smell.

Bring the motherfunking funk!

Vegetables aren't funky. Fuhrburger's diet—plant-based, avoiding oil, salt, sugar, and refined grains—don't bring da funk. It don't leave much dirty. My new diet was like fucking angels with Barney's autoclaved little dick.

You go out to a fancy restaurant and they bring a plate of funky cheese: smelly cow, sheep, and goat cheese. Cheese with some gooey brown paté with lumps of dirty, translucent fat in it. On the side are some weird-ass little pickles, and it's all sprinkled with pink rock salt. You eat that shit and know you're a grown-up. You know you're not really supposed to be eating that kind of stuff. Cheese is just food going bad. It's dirty, it's funky, it's gone bad, and you're eating it. That's sexy. That's not fucking a Barbie doll with a condom, that's barebacking a downtown hooker (maybe of your same sex) in a bathroom stall at a bus station. It's animal. It's sniffing butts and rolling in fuck. Take out all animal products, salt, sugar, and oil, and food is healthful and good but not funky at all.

Dr. Fuhrburger is not a funky guy. Pull out his book and look at him. Now pull out a P-Funk album and look at Bootsy Collins. Compare. My wife says the Fuhrburger recipes are a little like Boston Market. If you like one thing at Boston Market, you like everything at Boston Market, because it all tastes the same. You can tell a Fuhrburger recipe: it seems healthful and clean, and it doesn't make your dick stink.

I'm pretty far from Bootsy, but I have pissed in the next urinal down from where George Clinton was pissing (yes, of course I peeked, and no, I'm not publishing that info here. Ask me in person when I know you better). Dr. Funkenstein and I did a corporate show together back when dot-coms had all the money in the world and twenty-seven-year-old billionaires could say, "Let's have a corporate party with George Clinton and Parliament Funkadelic, Prince, and . . . and, oh, let's hire Penn & Teller to do some magic, too!"

I'm not Bootsy and I don't have to eat haggis, but I can't eat just plain carrots. I'm healthy and happy, but I need some food that reminds me of the way backstage at CBGB-OMFUG smelled in the '80s. Most adventurous eating, from stinky cheese to fish eyes to uni, is animal-based, so I needed to find a few things that could bring enough funk to get by.

Like mushrooms. Mushrooms can bring some funk. They grow in dirt and they aren't animals, but they can't make food from sunlight. Mushrooms grow in dark shit. Growing in dark shit is funky. And some of them look like aliens, and some of them look like penises. Some of them have weird pubic-hair-like cilia on them. You could fuck a mushroom, and it wouldn't be bad. They're not animals, but they are also not really plants. They are alien stuff. The biggest living thing in the world is a honey fungus that lives in the Blue Mountains of Oregon, if you call that living. Mushrooms live on dead things, and they reproduce with spores, not seeds. Mushrooms are funky, and mushrooms are fungus. "Fungus" sounds like "funky" and means funky. Mushrooms can psychedelicize your mind. Mushrooms can kill you, and that's funkier than Bootsy. That's Rick James. We put all kinds of mushrooms in everything. They give texture, sex, and flavor, and they always bring the funk. Mushrooms look like sex organs and burst with flavor, life, and health. There's a nut friend of CrayRay who has a different cult—some sort of mushroom cult—and he'll tell you mushrooms will cure cancer and get you hard and make you cum like a fire hose. I like them because they bring really different flavors and textures to my diet. One of the things I miss eating only plants is texture in food. Mushrooms give texture. Since I've been riding the CrayRay wagon, I've eaten a lot of mushrooms.

Then there's nutritional yeast; holy funk! There's another kingdom outside of plants that I eat. And it's also creepy. Nutritional yeast is neither plant nor animal. Yeast is even too weird to be fungus. Yeast is made up of creepy single cells smaller than plant and animal cells but bigger than bacteria. They have no chloroplasts, but their ribosomes are the same size as ours—like I said, creepy. I used to like eating stinky, disgusting, creepy cheeses and funky, creepy meats and fishes, and now I eat yeast and think about it being neither plant nor animal. You can't get funkier than yeast. Make sure you buy "nutritional yeast" and not just regular make-bread-rise or infectional yeast. Nutritional yeast is made to bring da funk and nothing else. They grow the little fuckers in molasses and then kill them dead, dead, dead. The kind of nutritional yeast you buy at AssWhole Foods has some added amino acids for the vegans, but Dr. Fuhrburger thinks added stuff is bad, so his brand doesn't have it. Doesn't matter; all the brands have da funk.

Most recipes tell you to use a spoonful or two of nutritional yeast here or there, but I keep it right on the table with the vinegar and the Tabasco, and I dump it on lots of stuff. When I was eating that great

corn/tomato stew over rice for my one meal every day, I would dump
so much nutritional yeast on that shit that it formed a powder floating on top like pond scum. Then I would let it soak a little and skim
it off. I wasn't eating stew with nutritional yeast, I was eating slightly
moist yeast. Can you think of a two-word phrase funkier than "moist
yeast"? I would dampen up my yeast with stew and beans and even
use it on my baked potatoes. I take a potato, bite off a hunk to expose
the virginal white potato flesh, sprinkle on some Tabasco to get that
baby hot and sticky, and then grind it into a pile of moist yeast. That
virginal potato is now fully wasted and ready to suck on down. Serious funk. Put a mess of mustard greens drenched in vinegar on the
side, and fuck that cheese plate with pickles in the neck. You've got a
good healthy funk.

So you've got whole plants and some funk thrown in, and a few
things that are kinda neither but maybe both:

SEASONINGS AND CONDIMENTS.

There's all this "Mrs. Dash" seasoning shit that's really good. There are
spicy ones and garlic ones, and they all add lots of flavor without any
salt. Fuhrburger also has a bunch of these, and we eat those, too. I love
it all and always use more than anyone else. I do not like moderation.
My wife buys all sorts of this stuff, and I just dump it on.

TABASCO.

Nothing compares to Tabasco. Hot sauce brings da funk. I once met
the great singer-songwriter Bonnie Raitt. We talked backstage at a
corporate show (not the same corporate show where I pissed next to
George Clinton—that would have been too gone even for the dot-
coms), and she had one piece of advice for me: "If you go to Russia,
bring Tabasco sauce."

CrayRay would like me to cut down on Tabasco, but I'm being

reprogrammed. I needed to take everything he said as gospel when I was a fat fuck, but now that I'm a bit more under control, I keep the salt out of my diet, but I take a grain with whatever CrayRay says. He thinks I should train myself to enjoy the natural taste of food a little more. Fuck him in the neck. I love Tabasco. Yup—it has salt in it. It has less salt than most other hot sauces, and my thinking is, if I can stand the burn, I get the reward of a little burst of salt. I put Tabasco on air-popped popcorn on MovieNight. I'm as happy with a bowl of beans and brown rice with Tabasco as with any other food. Right now, as I write this at the Starbucks in Harrah's Cherokee Casino Resort in North Carolina, I have three tiny "emergency" bottles of Tabasco that I get from room service at the Rio right here in my computer bag. Upstairs in my hotel room there's a normal-sized bottle in my luggage and a Tupperware container of it in the bag of potatoes and yams I brought from Vegas for my travel food (I eat potatoes plain on the airplane; I don't want to offend the other passengers with the strong smell and don't want to spill it, but it's there with me, ready to be thrown into the eyes of would-be terrorists). Backstage, as part of my travel kit, our stage manager, Burt, keeps a big bottle of Tabasco in her road box. Our travel rider, which the long-suffering Glenn sends out with our contracts, stipulates that my whole-plant-no-salt-no-sugar-no-oil backstage meal needs to be served to me with a full bottle of Tabasco. At home there's a bottle on the kitchen table, two more in the kitchen proper, and another in the home theater. We just moved into a house with a glassed-in, chilled wine rack area with places for five hundred bottles of wine. Our family are all teetotalers, so the plan is to fill that wine area with fresh herbs—but that takes time, so we just bought five hundred bottles of Tabasco and display them there. My buddy Doc Swan sends me a funny hot sauce brand every New Year's Day as a present, and I try many of them, but nothing has ever beaten Tabasco for me.

APPLE CIDER VINEGAR.

I like the hippie shit "with the mother," but I also like the strained and pasteurized stuff they sell at 7-Eleven. Balsamic vinegar and all the fruity (in both senses) ones are fine, but I always come back to apple cider. Fuhrburger suggests I eat lots of salads and steamed greens, and I love them all with vinegar. My mom always served boiled spinach with vinegar. Spinach with vinegar is a comfort food for me. I can't get enough vinegar. I like apple cider vinegar best. I bought stupid-expensive, they-saw-me-coming bottles of balsamic, aged for forty years in the genitals of nuns, and it wasn't better than plain, unpasteurized, New England hippie apple cider vinegar. The kind that's cloudy and has weird stuff floating in it. The kind that's funky. For many meals, I have three pounds of greens as my side dish. Can something be a side dish if it's bigger than your head? CrayRay's cult has made me crazy enough that spinach has become a junk food to me. It's not nutrient-heavy enough for me. The three pounds of boiled greens I have are swimming in vinegar. It doesn't matter what they are, so I might as well get healthier ones. I love collard greens, and love saying "collard greens." Kale is, of course, the trendy king of greens. Chard is great. And mustard greens have their own built-in funk. They'll give you a horseradish kick in the balls that goes really nicely with vinegar.

My mom also used to cut up radishes and cucumbers and put them in apple cider vinegar. Pickles can be really salty and aren't good for you, but just cutting up all kinds of vegetables and throwing them into apple cider vinegar makes them great. And funky. And intense. I dip steamed broccoli, cauliflower, and even squash in vinegar. I could dip my fluorescent LeBron sneakers in vinegar and gobble them down. You might want to go with some of those hoity-toity fig- or pecan-infused vinegars, but I like apple cider vinegar and keep it right on the table next to my Tabasco. Three pounds of boiled greens, shake on the Tabasco, and then dilute that with a shit-ton of apple cider vinegar. That's all I need to really feel like I've eaten something. Again, CrayRay would like me to enjoy the vegetables without adding a lot of flavor, but I've already fucked CrayRay in the neck; he's dead to me.

NUTS.

Nuts are good for me, and they are part of the diet, but I have to be careful not to just take handfuls all the time. I found out I could get fat on nuts. It's pretty easy to get a day's worth of calories just by eating some Louisiana pecans, even without the New England maple syrup. Even eating nuts sparingly, I still have to be careful. The SAD people are trying to fuck with my nuts. They roast them and add oil to them, even though the delicious little fuckers are already filled with oil and fat. We have to get our nuts at AssWhole Foods or somewhere like that to make sure there's no oil, roasting, or salt included in the deal. The exception is almonds. It's easy to find raw, plain almonds. When I'm at an airport sundry shop, the only thing I buy is almonds. They all have raw, unsalted almonds hanging right on the rack with the M&M's "trail mix." I love checking the ingredients. Even the airport almonds list on the package "Ingredients: Almonds." I like that. I buy a few packs and stick them in my computer bag in case I need a meal on the plane. It's a lot of calories, but they're very tasty and filling and so easy to transport and eat right out of the bag. I don't need utensils or even a napkin, and I don't have to bring down the tray table smeared with invisible virulent stranger snot.

My buddy Jason Garfield, the buff juggler, told me that Daesh live on almonds. Now, you know you can never trust a "friend of a friend" story, but this is a juggler-of-a-juggler story. There's no chance that this is true, but Jason says asshole-loser-nihilist-for-god terrorists live in caves and eat almonds. The *NYT* (not jugglers) seems to report that terrorists are often well educated and live in houses, so you go ahead and believe the "paper of record" over a couple of half-naked jugglers talking in the kitchen about nuts at 3:00 a.m., but I believe Jason, so with every almond I put in my mouth I think about taking that almond from the mouth of some fucking homicidal/suicidal, hateful piece of shit. Eating almonds is how a peacenik like me engages in the war against terror. "That's another bag of 'Irresistible Snacking,' 'Smart Eating,' 'Blue Diamond All-Natural Whole' almonds that won't go to the misunderstood-as-violent jihad." And I eat them on airplanes as an extra fuck-you to al-Qaeda!

I have to be very careful with the nuts, because I love all kinds of nuts so much. I like to come downstairs naked in the middle of the night when my willpower is low and have a few spoonfuls of peanut butter. It's rich people's peanut butter that's just peanuts—not roasted, no salt or oil added—but it still has a shit-ton of fat and calories. At 4:00 a.m. with my dick hanging out, I have no willpower, so my wife has to hide the nuts and the peanut butter from me.

Peanuts are pure truth. Tomatoes are sneaky. They're botanical fruits that are used as vegetables for cooking purposes. Chimpanzees are great apes that are referred to as monkeys for comedic purposes. Peanuts are *Leguminosae* that are enjoyed as nuts. Tomatoes and chimps fucked up and gave no hint of their linguistic cross-dressing in their name. Peanuts, however, lay it right out there. The peanut has a kind of honesty that tomatoes and chimps can't touch. It's a PEA-*that-we-eat-as-a*-NUT, and those words in the middle are silent. How much better would the world be if tomatoes were called "fruitveges" and chimpanzees were called "chimonkeys." That's a world where the terrorists wouldn't have a chance, even with me crawling around on the floor naked in the middle of the night trying to find where my wife hid the peanut butter instead of eating their almond supplies. One of the eating techniques I'm experimenting with is eating pistachios and other nuts out of the shell, so I have to take the time to crack them, but there are few things more luxurious for a guy my age than pistachio kernels already out of the shell and ready to eat by the handful. I'm old enough that when I was a child, pistachios were a rare and expensive treat. They were dyed that weird-ass red, and I would sit and eat them until my hands looked like Ted Bundy's (in terms of botany, pistachios aren't nuts, they're fruits—but I'm just going to let that go this time. You're welcome). My earliest memory of learning self-control and willpower was waiting until I'd opened a whole handful of pistachios before stuffing them into my mouth. I still use that memory to help my sexual prowess. If I only had nuts in the shell around, I would probably eat fewer of them—but what about my quality of life?

AVOCADOS.

I also have to be careful about avocados. If I can't find the peanut butter in the middle of the night, I'll settle for some guacamole. EZ makes it with a lot of cilantro, which keeps CrayRay and Goudeau out of it. But I have to be careful; guac and nuts can make me fat.

So, that's what I eat and don't eat on a regular basis. For holidays, "Rare and Appropriate," and when my daughter, Mox, asks me to take her out for ice cream, all bets are off. And it seems like once a year I like to eat just potatoes, but this'll tell you what I eat normally. That's what seems to keep me skinny and healthy. I didn't do it for flavor, I did it for health—but I now sincerely like the taste, smell, and texture of this stuff more than the shit I used to eat. Even with all the Tabasco, Mrs. Dash, and vinegar that I dump on things, there are still more different flavors than ever came through in pizza, steak, and spaghetti. The new diet is more interesting and exciting.

It took me a while to get here. That's the CrayRay genius. He does the cold-turkey potato thing to reset the taste buds, the smells, the habits, and the microbiome. None of this stuff would have tasted good a year ago. It didn't change, I did. It's still bland—I'm just more sensitive.

I guess this isn't the most attractive way to sell someone on this diet, but I'm not trying to sell you on this diet. I have no evidence that it's right for you, or even very much evidence that it's right for me. Maybe you want a little less funk and a little more apple tree. I'm just reporting on what I think happened with me and food. I keep thinking about *The Stranger* by Camus. He's writing about adjusting to prison and how he found a way to be content. I suppose it's a bit insensitive for me, as a free man, to compare eating healthy with being in prison while living in a country that uses jail to unjustly address too many social problems, so please take this with a grain of non-whole-plant salt as poetic and political. Yeah, Camus wrote it and not me, so fuck you. There's a passage where he writes: "As for the rest of the time, I managed quite well, really. I've often thought that had I been compelled to live in the trunk of a dead tree, with nothing to do but gaze up at the patch of sky just overhead, I'd have got used to it by degrees. I'd have learned to watch for the passing of birds or drifting clouds . . ."

When I had the whole world of American food at the tip of my tongue, it made me sick and I didn't enjoy it. Now that it's just whole plants, I enjoy every meal and I feel great. I see every cloud and every bird that passes by.

What do I eat? Whole plants. And please pass the funk.

"I LIKE FOOD TOO MUCH TO EAT LIKE YOU"

I've always prided myself on eating anything. It's a self-image change for me to now take time to explain to the waiter the stupid way I eat. I have to give detailed instructions for a salad, for Christ's sake. If I'm out with people and I don't want to be embarrassed by asking the staff whether the baked potatoes have any oil on the skin or some other stupid shit, I just order sparkling water and decaffeinated coffee and call that my supper. If I'm out with people at a restaurant, chances are I'm there for the company or business, and if I don't eat, it just makes focusing and talking easier. CrayRay has taught me that not eating at all is even an option, at least for a few weeks.

I have friends who have watched me get thin and healthy. They've watched me eat, even tasted what I eat. When they complain to me about their weight and their health and I say, "Just do what I did," they answer with something like "I like food too much to eat like you." To taste buds that have been fucked hard by the Standard American Diet, the food I now eat tastes bland at best, but to me it tastes great. To me it sounds a bit like they're saying, "I like music too much to listen to Miles Davis." It's not food you like too much, it's shitty, corporate, jive-ass, TV food you like too much.

What we eat and what we like to eat is completely habit. Every study I can find on it says people eat what they're used to eating and they like what they're told to like. When I started this diet, I thought I was going to go through three months without any good food—that I'd have food I loved only at "Rare and Appropriate" times, weeks apart. I was planning on giving up most of my food enjoyment, but I thought my health was worth it.

I didn't understand CrayRay's plan for me. His plan was to fix my broken palate. I now eat food I love every single day, at every single meal. And the food I love is more complex, more interesting, more jazz, classical, Velvet Underground, Zappa. It's just no shitty Eagles. I look forward to my meals more than I ever have, and when I finish my meal and I'm full, I don't feel slightly sick with my guts exploding. I feel great. It seems like human beings are going to grow to love whatever food we eat—we just have to learn to love the right foods and not eat what TV tells us to eat. As I said to one of my libertarian buddies, "Eating pizza is just voting for Hillary."

I'm from New England, and my parents were a generation older than all my peers' parents. My mom fed me delicious, well-prepared, healthful food made with care and love. I didn't eat shitty snacks. Yeah, there was way too much of all the stuff I don't eat now, but my mom didn't know. I loved the food my mom served me because I loved my mom and I was used to it. When I left home as a teenager, there was a lot of exploring and learning to do, and a small part of that experimenting was trying food that wasn't offered in Greenfield.

When I arrived in Frisco in my twenties, some new friends took me out for sushi. When I worked with George Takei and became friends with him, he claimed that he was responsible for sushi being so popular in the USA. He says he took William Shatner out for sushi on the set of *Star Trek*, and there you go. I remain a little skeptical, but I'm always a little skeptical. In the late '70s sushi was still exotic outside of California, and I'd never had it. I wasn't a sci-fi fan. I sat down at the counter and my friends explained that we'd start with a "California roll" because it was "easy for beginners." Fuck that. I called the sushi chef over and asked, "What do people who look like me never order?"

It didn't take long for him to size me up. He answered, "Uni."

"Okay, my friends and I will have nothing but uni, a big plate of it. However many orders that is."

He explained that it was sea urchin and it had a taste and texture we wouldn't be used to and it was expensive. I was a street performer and had plenty of cash. As long as he was okay being paid in ones, I'd gladly treat all my buddies to *Star Trek: The Supper*. We had a feast of uni, and, wow, it was weird. My boiled-dinner-New-England-palate had no idea what hit it. This was not corned beef and cabbage. I've enjoyed sushi ever since that day, but I faded back to California rolls, and it was a few years before I got back into uni.

I was a judge on some Food Network cooking show, and the contest was preparing the most expensive foods. I ate Kobe beef that was six hundred bucks for one steak *before* it was prepared, and the freshest, rarest, most delicate sea urchins. I was grown up and could dig all those flavors. I'd come a long way from New England.

Now I've come even farther from New England. I've lost my taste for doughnuts, pizza, and bacon. I never thought it would be possible. I thought the love of grease, sweet, and salt was built in. I had lots of just-so stories that explained it from an evolutionary standpoint. Calories and salt were scarce, and we had to look for all we could get. It doesn't seem that way now. I order organic, vegan soup at a health food store, and it's just too salty for me to finish. In the old days, I would have pushed through. In the old days, as a fat fuck, I would have ignored the chemical burn of the salt and kept eating until the recoil turned to desire. I would push through the waxy phony taste of a Hershey bar because TV told me it was a treat. Vote for Hillary because she's the sane choice. I learned to love the sea urchin. I don't do that anymore. I've worked hard to get my palate to where it is. I don't show off anymore by being able to enjoy eating anything. I don't have to use that to show off—I have a theater with my name on it and I can vanish a cow dressed as an elephant.

I'm writing this at Christmastime. Because I have my name on a theater, my bosses at the Rio All-Suite Hotel and Casino in Las Vegas, Nevada, always get me a present for the holidays. They learned years ago that they were fucked on the alcohol front, that they'd booked the only teetotalers in showbiz. They couldn't just buy a nice bottle of something and be done with it. They solved that problem with food. Every Christmas they give me a huge basket of all sorts of delicacies. This year I went through the basket pretty quickly. Not eating—sorting. Chocolates, salty toffee nuts, olives, tapenade, gourmet shortbreads, and ginger cookies all went to our crew. I took home a few pieces of fresh fruit. This is fancy fresh fruit, big perfect oranges and apples and some plums.

I've never enjoyed eating more than I do right now. I love pea soup, beans, salad, and fresh watermelon more than I ever enjoyed Kobe beef and uni.

So, my answer to my friends' statement is "I now like food too much to eat like you."

TIME TRAVEL

The day I started eating only potatoes, I started taking pictures of myself every morning. I'm a shitty photographer, but right after I weighed myself, right before my shower, I banged out about twenty pictures in the bathroom mirror. I continued that every day until I hit my target weight eighty-six days later. I just snapped pictures as I turned my fat ass in the mirror. I took 1,648 pictures in my underwear between December 9, 2014, and March 5, 2015. I pushed hard for this book to be a flip-book, but Simon & Schuster wanted words and shit. If movies hadn't been invented by a frog magician, this here magician would have invented them right now, and The Man would have stepped on that, too. But you take your own pictures, mount them in your own little book, and riffle one way and you lose weight, and riffle the other and you go back to being a fat fuck right before your eyes. That's what I do with pictures in the privacy of my home. Magic.

I wasn't planning on doing a book when I first started taking these pictures. I was just planning to eat potatoes and try to stay out of the hospital. I didn't need pictures to keep track of my weight loss—I had my magic Withings scale, which not only kept track of every tenth of a pound but also ratted me out instantly to CrayRay. He still gets my weight sent to him every time I step on the scale. Maybe I should have it sent to L. Ron Hubbard, too.

I tell all my friends who want to ease on down the CrayRay road that they should take a lot of pictures. And they should take them as close to naked as possible. There are way too many pictures of me already. I have professional photo shoots all the time, and people snap a few hundred pictures of me every night after our show. I am well documented, but I still wanted underwear shots every morning during my rapid weight loss so I could go back and watch it later.

The future is here, man. We still dream about time travel, but we already have it, and it's getting better all the time. The usual science fiction rules for time travel are that you can go back in time and see and hear everything, but you can't do anything to change it. That's a pretty good definition of video. Now there's video of everything all the time, but even back when I was little, my brother-in-law had a super-8 camera (my sister was much older than me), and I have some video of me as a preteen running around with my family. I don't watch it often, but when I do, it gives me the exact sweet melancholy I would expect from time travel, but I can't kill Hitler or buy Microsoft.

With everyone carrying a full studio with them all the time in their phones, people in the real future are going to be able to re-create whole cities by merging together GPS- and time-stamped pictures and video from our time. They will all be able to virtually travel to Disney World at any second of the past and watch it stay exactly the same.

I worry a little about the young adults of today. I worry that they aren't sexting quite enough and won't have enough naked pictures and porn video of themselves. I worry there's still too much false information about society's unnecessary stigma about sex. There's stuff in the news all the time about college students sexting, but still reports say that fewer than half of young adults are sexting pictures of themselves. I don't want to see pictures of young people naked. I'm old and I'm creepy, but I'm not that creepy. What I want is pictures of my friends and myself when we were twenty. I want just what at least half of young people are going to have when they themselves are old and creepy. The news sources I read (which are for old people like me) fret about young adults not understanding that when they post nude pictures of themselves, those pictures will never go away. That's a feature, not a bug, and fortunately at least half of young adults know that. As David Bowie sang, "And these children that you spit on / They're quite aware of what they're going through / Ch-ch-ch-ch-changes." Have you been a hung American?

Even if that low scare number of "almost 50 percent" of young adults sexting pictures is accurate (I think and hope it's much higher), it means that within forty years we'll have a Supreme Court justice with youthful sex pictures on the web. Old people worry that these pictures will come back to haunt them and ruin careers. What they don't seem to realize is that there's a better way to solve this issue, a way that doesn't involve fewer sex pictures. It's the sane way. Society can simply stop punishing people for being sexual. We're working on solving the problem of people being punished for gay sex not by teaching people to be sneakier about the gay sex they're having but rather by society accepting gay sex. We can solve the problem of people ruining others' lives with nude and sex pictures of them by society deciding not to ruin people's lives for nude and sex pictures. Society needs to decide that nude and sex pictures are good things, not bad things. That's the future.

"Remember when that nude photo of Hillary Clinton at Yale turned up? Remember that made the news?"

"Goofy."

The members of my generation who consider nude pictures a bad thing will be dead soon (that's not a threat, that's just time; the members of my generation who think they're a good thing will also be dead soon). The kids are alright. I'm a little too old to have great nude pictures and video of myself when I was twenty years old. I have a few Polaroids, but not enough. I have a picture of myself at about twenty in cutoff shorts (as close as I got to Daisy Dukes), and I just love it. I'm a young, healthy hippie with hair down my back, a big smile, and a happy bulge in my jeans and none at my waist. I like to travel back to that time now and again.

In the early mid-'90s I went to see genius actor/comedian/writer/buddy of mine Paul Provenza in a production of genius actor/comedian/writer/musician/buddy of mine Steve Martin's play *Picasso at the Lapin Agile*. After the play I was invited out with a bunch of people to have a cup of coffee and talk. I happened to sit down next to a beautiful woman, maybe about fifty years old. I introduced myself, and she introduced herself as Xaviera Hollander, the "Happy Hooker." I'm exactly the right age to know that name immediately, even without the honorific, but to make sure, she reached into her purse, pulled out her wallet, and showed me a nude picture of herself at about twenty years old. "That's what I looked like," she said proudly. I have trouble telling this story with the right tone. I've told it to a lot of friends, and they see it as desperate, sad, even pathetic. I don't know how to make clear it wasn't like that. It was beautiful. She still looked great sitting next to me, and she showed me the picture with a big smile and a wink. She seemed happy with how she looked now, but she showed me a picture of an earlier her. It was one of the grooviest introductions I've ever gotten. I was a little embarrassed that I couldn't whip out a photo of my own and show her me naked at the same age. I was the one who was desperate, sad, and even pathetic because I did *not* have a picture. I deflected by bragging that I had an original pressing of her LP *Xaviera!*

I loved her sex stories on that record, and I even liked her version of the Beatles' "Michelle" and her duet with Ronnie Hawkins. Now that we'd broken the ice, I busted her. On the recording, I think in the Hawkins duet, she had a line that I remembered as "Whoever said 'all men are created equal' never saw Bo Diddley in the shower." I was not going to take issue with Xaviera about the size of Bo Diddley's cock. Even Christopher Hitchens couldn't have won that argument. But I did think that she could have credited Thomas Jefferson with the "All men are created equal" thing. When I look it up, the web remembers it as a Ronnie Hawkins line that goes "Abraham Lincoln said all men are created equal, but he never saw Bo Diddley coming out of the shower." Now, I'm willing to bet that Abraham Lincoln did say that, but I bet Abe credited Thomas Jefferson. Neither Abe nor Tom ever saw Bo Diddley coming out of the shower. Maybe Ronnie and Xaviera just didn't want to open that Jefferson-was-a-slave-owner can of worms. That led me to doing schtick for Xaviera about how Elvis Presley during the chatter section of "Are You Lonesome Tonight?" says, "You know, someone said that all the world's a stage. And each must play a part . . ." It wasn't "someone" who said that, it was Shakespeare, you hillbilly piece of shit! But of course when Jolson recorded it years earlier, he couldn't bring Shakespeare to mind, either, and Al wasn't a hillbilly, he was from Lithuania. Thomas, William, and Abe certainly never saw Bo come out of the shower. I met Mr. Diddley, but not in the shower. I can't speak to what Xaviera and Elvis might have seen of Bo, but she had great nude pictures of herself, and I sure hope there are some nudes of Elvis somewhere. He looked pretty different at twenty than at forty-two.

My buddy Bob Corn-Revere is a real, no-kidding First Amendment attorney. I love him. Bob was staying at my house in Vegas, and we were chatting about John Stagliano, known in professional porn as Buttman. Bob was following John's obscenity case and wanted to meet him. I had met John a couple of times, so I called him up and we all went out to supper together. Bob one-upped Xaviera. John was considering putting Bob on his legal team and asked Bob if he had a résumé. Bob said something like, "It's probably easier to just go to the Supreme Court website and pull up some of the audio of my arguments there." Yeah, Bob. That beats twenty-year-old naked pictures of yourself looking like Debbie Harry. We were talking about John's case. He had put out videos on the web that some crazy person in the Justice Department (who probably doesn't have pictures of himself naked at twenty) thought were obscene. Whiskey Tango Foxtrot?! It was milk enemas or something. This was the cheesy hill on which the US government wanted to die. I was just listening to Bob talk about the legal points, but during the conversation John mentioned that there was really very little money left in porn. Actors in porn used to make a lot of money, but although demand had gotten higher, supply had exceeded it. There wasn't a lot of dough-re-me. One could make pretty much the same money steaming soy milk at Starbucks as squirting it out of one's ass on camera. I asked Buttman, "Why do the actors do it, then?" John's answer stuck with me: "I think they want to immortalize their youth."

I have a friend. She's in her thirties. She's wicked smart and a very successful lawyer (I like lawyers). The day she turned eighteen she was in an Ivy League college setting the groundwork for law school. She was doing well, and was known among her friends for being rather prudish. She wasn't a party person; she liked to study. A couple of weeks before she turned eighteen, she searched around the web (I guess she wasn't too distracted by Buttman's milk videos), and found one of those "Barely Legal"–type sites that features naked men and women who have recently hit the age of consent. Without anyone knowing (I found out much later, and I'm one of the few who knows), she got in touch with a pornographer and said she wanted to model. They offered her a few grand, and she had to get them a lot of paperwork

FOOD IS GOD

My buddy and *Penn's Sunday School* cohost Matt Donnelly lost a shit-ton of weight right after I did. He looks like a new person. He needed to go even below his high school weight because he was already a fat fuck in high school. He's now way below his high school weight. He's the lightest he's been as an adult. It's a big deal. He did comedy with a lot of fat guy material. He lost a lot of his act along with the weight. Weight changes performance. Matt does improv with his partner, Paul Mattingly, and their style has changed. They used to be two fat guys stuck dealing with each other, but now Matt has to treat Paul differently. He can still bust his balls and condescend to him, but now Matt has to play the bad guy more often. If Matt attacks Paul directly, the audience turns on Matt. Now Matt is kind of the wiseass, the ballsy kid who gets kicked out of class. The body changes content and style.

I used to be able to stand onstage and have a certain kind of power just standing there like a monolith. Now I have to replace some of that weight with energy. I move more. It's a big change. Matt could to prove she really was of age. She set up a nude shoot for the week of her birthday. She met the photographer in his studio, and they took hundreds of pictures. She had done the arithmetic and figured that without her name out there (and it wasn't), no one would ever be able to find those pictures to use against her even if she ended up having the legal career she's having. That was decades ago, and there has been no downside. She's thrilled that she immortalized her youth.

I have a son who is nine years old and a daughter who is ten. I will not tell them to take nude pictures of themselves when they reach adulthood. I will not tell them to sext. As a matter of fact, we will reinforce all the stuff the schools tell them about being careful about information on the web. It's still a new thing and it's full of exaggerated dangers, but they're still dangers. Society has not hit the point where everyone they will ever work for will be okay with sexual pictures. They have to be careful, and I will explain that to them. But if they're listening carefully (and I have no evidence they have ever listened to me carefully), they might notice that while I'm telling them to be very careful . . . I'm not telling them not to do it. I'm not sure they should put milk up their asses on camera, but they might want to find a private way to immortalize their youth.

I have turned this chapter around. I started out writing about how I wanted to time travel to when I was a fat fuck to see my progress, and now I'm making the opposite point about using pictures to immortalize youth.

Yup—I'm glad I have pictures of myself when I started this diet, and I wish I had pictures of myself at twenty getting a milk enema.

Because that would be a great flip-book.

be meaner when he was fatter. He needed to be in a big fat glass house if he wanted to throw stones. In comedy, thin people have to be kinder. The thinner me is much nicer, offstage and on. I smile more onstage. It's not just that I feel better, although that's part of it. It's not just that I'm happier, although that's part of it. It's also that I can feel that the audience wants this thinner me to be different. Not only do movements look different on a thinner me but also ideas are understood differently. I have to do a little bit of massaging of how I present the message because the medium has changed.

Matt's stand-up and improv have changed, and he auditions for different TV and movie roles. He's no longer the belching, pizza-stained, rude friend or the creepy goofball in the diaper. He's now the regular guy, maybe even a leading man; I guess we'll see. His wife dated him fat. She married him fat. She fucked him fat. Now he's a thin guy, and better-looking than she bargained for. It's the same for my wife. This is the thinnest she's ever seen me, and that's nutty, but I'm not as good-looking as Matt. I'm sure his wife, Sarah, doesn't really love him any more now than she did before, but things sure didn't get worse when he got better-looking. They both claim to me that they enjoy fucking more now that Matt is skinnier, but they haven't demonstrated that to me yet; maybe if he (or I) loses a few more pounds. Matt and Sarah have two little babies, and when Matt was a sick, fat fuck, he had to really push to help care for them. Now he's getting off his meds, and he has more energy for his family. The new Matt is better for Matt and for his family.

Matt is also embracing the vanity that my New England upbringing won't let me celebrate full-on. Maybe it's not the New England–New Jersey difference between us; maybe it's just that he's better-looking than me. He looks great in his new skinny suits, and he knows it. When Matt was fat he landed the understudy part of Christian Grey in the live musical parody of *50 Shades of Grey* here in Vegas.

It's written for a fat guy in the lead. There's a bunch of fat jokes. There are dance numbers in which Christian wears nothing but a tiny red singlet—one of those Borat banana-hammock mankini things that just barely slings over the cock and balls and then goes up over the shoulders. Matt thought he might lose his job with the weight loss, but god is kind, and even thin guys look appalling in red singlets. Speaking of god, Matt said to me after he'd hit his target weight, "It's just atheism. It's all just atheism."

It *is* all just atheism, and since I've written two books that were supposed to be about atheism (while actually being more about dropping my cock into a blow-dryer) the way this book is supposed to be about losing weight (but might as well be about dropping my cock in a blow-dryer), it seems I should explain. I'm going to guess from the people I see at my book signings that many people who will read this book are atheists who also might feel that they need to lose weight. I'll do my best to tie those two things together.

Christopher Hitchens argued that everyone is atheist about almost all gods—full atheists just go one god further. Everyone knows what it feels like to not believe in Thor; one just has to extend that peaceful easy feeling one god further.

Many people reading this book already know what it feels like to live in a culture where everyone takes things for granted that aren't true. As Bob Dylan sang, "To live outside the law, you must be honest." Yup—being honest and living outside the law are all it takes to be thin.

I'm a big-ass capitalist. I'm all for food companies and drug companies and doctors doing anything they can to honestly sell their services and get as rich as they can. Our bodies are not their responsibility—our bodies are our own responsibilities. It should not take a village to decide what I eat. People with something to sell should tell the truth and shouldn't cheat, but they are not responsible for my personal decisions. And it's my responsibility to be informed about my decisions. That's all me, not them, and it sure shouldn't be the guys with the guns collecting taxes.

The government should not ban cigarettes or trans fats, but just because they're legal doesn't mean I should use them. It's not the government's responsibility to keep me healthy. I don't get pissed at lobbyists for rigging the diet game on package labeling, I get pissed at people for thinking the government should help them eat right. I'm not talking reality (am I ever?). In reality, the government makes us pay in all sorts of ways for everyone else's health care, so everything you do in the United States really is my business. It's my financial business. Once we've set up the government to force people to pay for one another's healthcare, freedom goes out the window. If I'm paying even indirectly for your healthcare, you are not smoking or riding that motorcycle, young lady. And how much of my money gets put at risk every time you take it bareback up the ass, young man? It's some of my money, so why don't you take all those sexy men out of your bedroom and go see a movie, and wear a seatbelt, or better yet, walk there . . . in the afternoon . . . on the sidewalk . . . wearing a fluorescent orange vest . . . and a hard hat, when there's no lightning and no heart-clogging popcorn for anyone ever!

If you want to be a fat fuck, you should be able to be a fat fuck as long as I don't have to pay for your hypertension, diabetes, heart problems, colon cancer, and all the other shit that's probably more likely to strike you at your fat-fuck weight. It should be an individual decision. I don't know what's best for other people. Did Jim Morrison have a better life than me being killed by drugs before he was half my age? I don't know. I really don't know. Orson Welles and Marlon Brando: did they enjoy eating more than they would have enjoyed making more brilliant art? I don't know.

McDonald's is going to work hard to sell you shitty food—salt, sugar, and fat that we all know is bad for us. Okay. Lots of people are trying to sell you shitty music and shitty movies and shitty religions. Churches are trying to sell you on wasting your life and misplacing your love. As long as we don't subsidize the fructose that McDonald's sells or give the churches a tax break, I'm fine with all that. I know we already do those things, but for the sake of argument let's pretend we don't. Let's push for freedom. I want to be free to not smoke marijuana and not do heroin. I'm not really free to not do anything if it's illegal. I don't get credit. It's more fun to not eat trans fats and fructose if they are legal and everywhere. I want the power to honestly choose for myself not to do something. Being an atheist is its own kind of special fun in a Christian nation. "To live outside the law, you must be honest."

I'm writing personally about "fun." It's been fun for me in this Christian nation. I've been treated very well by Christians, and I've been able to laugh at the goofiness, but I'm aware that it was anything but fun for many of the atheist heroes in this country who paved the way for the rest of us and who were persecuted for their lack of faith. Madalyn Murray O'Hair had her family beaten almost to death. That sure wasn't fun.

And there are lots of insults that aren't much more than a little pain in the ass in the big picture but still aren't fun. An atheist friend of mine had a ten-inch (don't get excited) blood clot in his neck that was killing him, and the doctor told his wife it was because they were atheists. That's appalling, but really, without the stroke symptoms they could have laughed it off. Their suffering on that night (he got better; I guess prayer does work) had pinned the pain VU meter, so the Christ-loving asshole MD didn't really make it any worse.

My daughter didn't have fun when a classmate told her in third grade that her family's being atheist meant that her mom and dad didn't love her. We confronted the kid's parents, and they explained that they weren't even religious. They had no idea where that bullying came from, but we all know where the bullying came from: it came from the buzz-kill Christian nation. It's not all fun.

I am a big fan of the anonymous avant-garde music/art/performance group the Residents. I weaseled my way into working with them, so I got to watch their fans get very sad when the band had any success at all, because part of what their fans love about the music is that not everyone loves the music. There are some who think that *Mamma Mia!* on Broadway must be good because it's successful, and others who think it must be bad because it's successful. I think it must be bad because of ABBA.

It was so stupid that I would revel in being an outsider, a teetotaling, Residents-loving atheist in a drunken, Céline Dion–loving, Christian nation, yet still eat exactly what that same culture was telling me to eat. I was all bacon and doughnuts, pretending that I was rebelling against the food scolds when really I was just getting down on my knees and praying to the big fat status quo while Canadians sang pablum.

I was so good at sitting smugly in a restaurant and watching everyone else order expensive wines and get stupid, and yet I was putting multiple pats of butter on every piece of hot processed bread, putting salt on my prime rib before I tasted it, putting extra blue cheese dressing on my salad, and preordering the chocolate soufflé that took an extra twenty minutes to prepare. That was not thinking for myself. That was buying the hype all the way. I was raised in the Church of Food, and I was a believer—yeah, I was a believer.

It's pretty easy to see why. I was never a Christian as an adult. I wasn't part of that cult. I never smoked dope or drank liquor. I'd been to a church without faith, I'd been to a Dead concert without drugs, and I'd been to Gilley's country bar (the real one in Texas with David Allen Coe playing, not the Vegas one with pop-country) without liquor. I knew what it looked like to watch that mass insanity from my sober, rational high horse. But my mom fed me tender pork roast with delicious, salty gravy, and I never thought the Clash singing "You must not act the way you were brought up" applied to that. I had eaten more than half a dozen glazed, raspberry-filled Krispy Kreme doughnuts at one sitting. I'd stuffed my face with chicken and waffles. I got my hot fudge sundaes with extra hot fudge, and my bacon and eggs with extra bacon and eggs and a double order of buttered white toast. In the food department, I was shooting china white and talking in tongues.

I considered the people who were telling me this food was bad for me to be hippies or scolds. I never had a fun person tell me to eat sane. Nobody fun ever told me I was eating myself to death. I didn't want to eat sane. I say proudly that I don't ever do recreational drugs. I don't ever drink. It's pretty clear that if I was going to have a toke, if I was going to shoot heroin, if I was going to sip wine with dinner, I'd end up like Charles Bukowski, and if I opened up my heart to Jesus, I'd be evangelical. I'm an all-or-nothing kind of guy. I'm sickened by what my buddy Debbie Harry described in song as cases of "partial extremes." The kind of guy I am, if I couldn't eat nothing, I was going to eat everything.

There is nothing fun and sexy about moderation. To be thin, I needed to find a way to make my diet as extreme as my other lifestyle choices. I didn't want to be half-assed. Sometimes when talking about my new diet, I just say, "I don't eat." When I met Charlie Brooker, the genius behind *Black Mirror*, in England, we were making plans for lunch and he said, "I don't know where to go; you just eat vegetables rolled in chocolate, right?" I said, "Not exactly; I eat twigs rolled in chocolate and dirt, but I can eat that anywhere." I really don't need a diet that allows me to fit in. I'm fine going to a place that serves meat, cheese, oil, salt, liquor, and methamphetamines and plays ABBA, but I'm still going to just have a plain nothing-but-plants salad with no dressing except vinegar on the side—or I can eat nothing. Eating nothing is the option I never had before. It doesn't work for a year or really even for a month, but it sure works for a supper meeting.

When people are going out for a heavy Standard American Diet meal, I don't want to say, "I eat carefully," so I say, "I don't eat." Fasting is so much sexier than ordering carefully. It's a lie, but I like lies sometimes.

Now I don't drive through fast food joints, I drive by them, just like I drive right past the bars and the churches and Céline Dion. These are parts of my culture that are not for me. I'm a cat who simply doesn't go to those places. So many of my previous diets tried to make it easy for me, to make me fit in while dieting. What I'm doing now makes me a creep, and I like being a creep. It's so much easier than partial extremes. I was always an outsider to a lot of hype; I just finally lost faith in one hype further. If Hitchens were alive (and he might be if he hadn't drunk, smoked, and eaten badly), I think he might understand. I've just given up one god more. It's just atheism. I must not act the way I was brought up.

I watch movies and TV in which people pray, drink, toke, and eat, and these aren't movies about me. I don't want movies about me. I want movies about the dead coming back to earth and guys who can blow themselves. Why do I want to see a movie about me? I *am* me.

On my favorite John Lennon album, *The Plastic Ono Band*, made right after he stopped being brought down by the Beatles and finally did his best work with his wife, Yoko Ono (yup—I'm very comfortable with the outsider position), he has a song called "God." It starts with the line "God is a concept by which we measure our pain"—the usual John Lennon writing that sounds wicked heavy and doesn't really mean very much. The kind of writing that I really like. After that empty intro, he just starts repeating the phrase "I don't believe in . . ." and then ends every line with a different thing he doesn't believe in, like Buddha, Jesus, Yoga, Gita, Zimmerman (we could fight over that one, but someone already shot him), and so on. He ends the list with "I don't believe in . . . Beatles." I've loved that song since I was a child. My hero, the Amazing Randi, had The Amaz!ng Meeting in Las Vegas with zillions of skeptics and atheists, and at my private party for them, my band, the NoGodBand, did a cover of "God," but when we got to the "I don't believe in . . ." section, we just passed the mic around the audience for a while and let people yell out things they didn't believe in: "dousing," "ESP," "UFOs," "Muhammad," "chiropractors"—the list went on and on until the band got tired. Skinny Penn would now add to that list "animal products," "refined grains," "salt," "sugar," and "oil."

John Lennon then ends the song with "I just believe in me / Yoko and me / and that's reality."

Diet is just atheism. I just believe in me / plants and me / and that's reality.

The dream is over.

TV COOKING

Can I still write light, good-natured, fun stuff about my stints on *The Celebrity Apprentice*, even though we now know that one of my costars, Donald Trump, would one day fill our country with embarrassment, hate, and fear? Is this going to feel like a cute little anecdote about Kristallnacht? This isn't about Trump, it's about food, diet, us, and me; fuck Trump in the neck.

What the other "celebrities" on *The Celebrity Apprentice* hated about the show (besides Trump) was doing stuff they didn't know how to do. What I loved about doing the show was doing stuff I didn't know how to do. I'm very comfortable with that. Maybe "comfortable" isn't the right word. "Happy" may be the right word. I'm very happy doing things I don't know how to do, and that's fortunate for me, because I don't know how to do very much. My job in *The Penn & Teller Show* is doing things we don't know how to do. Teller always points out that a musician learns how to play piano, and once that's done, she can play a zillion songs and keep learning new ones on the same instrument, building new art on top of her basic skill set. With magic, it's different. The skills necessary to perform a new bit are, for the most part, different from any skills we've ever used before, and it's unlikely we'll ever use them again. Sure, I have experience talking on-stage, and Teller has experience acting onstage, and those are transferable. We have an idea of what the audience is likely to go along with and enjoy, and that skill is evergreen. And most important, we're both fabulous liars, but tricks need to be created and learned new. It's as if every time we want to play a new song, we have to invent the instruments and then learn to play them. When Teller and I are working on new material, every week we get to do something we've never done before, and it's not uncommon for that something to be something no one has ever done before. I love it.

So, doing something I'd never done before on a silly TV show was a blast. Other contestants would brag that something was right in his or her "wheelhouse," but I was happiest when no one had any idea how to do something. I want to do the shit I don't know how to do. I want to learn. This extends to other "reality" shows as well. I used to think that if I wanted to put asses in Penn & Teller Theater seats, my TV appearances had to be about doing magic. And if the spot wasn't about magic, it should at least be funny. And if it wasn't funny or magic, the two of us should at least be wearing our matching gray suits. Or if it was just me alone wearing jeans, I should at least be in my loud, aggressive *Bullshit!* character. It seems that's just not true at all. I can go on TV pretty much as myself, not in P&T drag, and be thoughtful and polite with no tricks or jokes, and it still brings people to our show. Once we learned that, we could say yes to all sorts of things that had nothing to do with our show and still sell tickets. Lots more chances to do things I have no idea how to do.

There's a cooking show called *Rachael vs. Guy*. Rachael Ray and Guy Fieri each captain a celebrity team for a cooking competition.

It was much gentler, kinder, and fairer than *The Celebrity Apprentice* and didn't star someone who is mentally ill, but it was the same idea. The producers called and asked if I cooked. The long-suffering Glenn explained that of course I cooked and I'd love to go on. Glenn has also learned to lie in his job. He then called me and said, "Penn, you've got a couple of weeks to learn to cook."

EZ found me Jet Tila, a world-class chef and a world-class guy. Jet agreed to come to Vegas for a few days and spend some hours with me teaching me how to cook for reality TV shows. Our goal was very specific. I was not going to learn to cook for my family and myself. I was not going to learn to cook at a restaurant. I was not going to learn to be a chef. I was not going to learn nutrition or home economics. I was going to learn to cook on TV and win. On reality TV competition shows, there are always at least two competitions going on. There's the competition that's the make-believe of the show, and there's the real competition that happens outside the TV show. Winning the make-believe competition does help with winning the real competition, but they're not the same. Let's take, for example, Piff the Magic Dragon.

Piff is now a very close friend on mine, but the first time I saw him, he was competing against me on a show called *Penn & Teller: Fool Us*. The show's premise is this: a magician comes out and does a trick for Penn & Teller, and if we know how the trick is done, the magician loses. If we don't know how the trick is done, if the magician fools us, he or she wins. We're pretty proud of the central idea of the show. Teller and I both hate shows that have some supposedly omnipotent judge who rules capriciously on behalf of entertainment. I can't watch *American Idol* because all I can think about is how poorly Bob Dylan, Tiny Tim, and Sun Ra would do on that show, while mediocre dipshits spewing nonsense about art are successful. Fuck them all. We get around that in *FU* by not talking about anything except the very personal and specific question of

"Were we fooled?" It's very clear that the best trick might not fool us, and the worst trick might fool us. We're just judging that one very personal thing. Did we feel fooled?

Piff came on *FU* and killed. The crowd could not have loved him more. We could not have loved him more. His attitude and his comedy were perfect, and his trick was amazing. He blew the audience away. Everyone, including us, jumped to our feet in applause and screamed for Piff. He destroyed. But Piff lost. He lost the make-believe competition. We happened to figure out how the trick was done (or we thought we did; since having become friends with Piff and having a lot of discussion, it's a bit less clear. In retrospect, he might have actually fooled us), and he lost. His YouTube clip of the show got millions of hits, his career took off, one thing led to another, and he was on *America's Got Talent*, where he also lost with the jive-ass judges but won the real contest, and now he's very successful and tours all over and makes a shit-ton of money. Piff is an example of losing the pretend game and winning the real game. "In the final end he won the wars after losing every battle," as Bob sang.

Adam Carolla did the same thing on *The Celebrity Apprentice*. He didn't get far—Trump threw him off for a really unfair and stupid reason (that was Trump's job)—but at the end of the season, Adam was more respected and loved by the audience than my buddy who won, Arsenio Hall. Jet would teach me to go on a TV cooking show and do my best to win the make-believe competition, but also have the style and confidence to win the real competition and put those asses in P&T Theater seats.

The first lesson was quite something. He told me very simply that the way he was teaching me to cook would get me fired from any restaurant and make my family sick, but it could win on TV. I would cook with more salt, oil, and sugar than even I could believe. Every mouthful the judges ate would be dripping with fat, sugar, and salt.

Even by the standards of what I was eating then—and this was at my worst—the way Jet was teaching me to cook was appalling. I can't emphasize enough that Jet is a great cook for reals. Jet knows nutrition. Jet knows health. Jet knows subtle, complex flavors. When my eating changed and I'd have suppers for friends, Jet loved and understood the new food. He loved eating it and could prepare it perfectly. Jet could have taught me how to cook to be as thin and healthy as I am now, but back then, right before *Rachael vs. Guy*, that wasn't his job. He was teaching me to cook on TV. Butter, olive oil, coconut oil, fry oil, vats of oil, Kobe beef, chicken wings, cream, brown sugar, maple sugar, more sugar, some sour and fat to cut it a bit, more sugar, kosher salt, Himalayan pink rock salt, handfuls of salt to distract from the fat and sugar and to work with the fat and sugar, salt and sugar, fat and salt, and sugar and fat and salt and fat and sugar and salt. He taught me knife skills, which are just juggling, so I loved those. And juggling swirling, flipping pans. He told me to make up a story with every dish. If I was cooking a Thai dish, I would make sure I told the judges that my grandmother, right off the boat from Thailand, taught me this dish, and it reminds me of my youth in Chiang Mai.

Because Vegas is the happiest place on earth, some strip clubs contain gourmet restaurants, and EZ sent me to Sapphire to work with a great chef, Jamaal Taherzadeh, who created my "favorite dish," Halibut Casino. This was just for TV. I would need a favorite dish, and I needed to remind people that Penn & Teller played Vegas. Halibut Casino would be perfect; I would cook it for the finale and just alibi the assignment to make it fit. Jet taught me to cook exactly five things and told me to just find a way to explain how one of those fit any assignment. It was just improv skills. Storytelling to fit, for instance, my Thai peg into a Hawaiian hole. It's pretty clear on the show that I'm doing that; we get the assignment and everyone else tries to plan a menu that follows the rules, while I mentally go through my five dishes, pick the best one, and then start jiving to make it seem like I just invented it.

Jamaal invented and taught me to make Halibut Casino in one afternoon in the kitchen of Sapphire while the topless pool was in full swing. I was chopping and sautéing while friendly topless women in thongs were leaning in to see what was going on and asking us for little tastes. If anyone ever tells you that I have a hard job, you can disabuse them of that notion in a hurry. And remember, my wife set this up. If anyone tells you that someone has a better life partner than me, you can disabuse them of that as well. I was surrounded by beautiful topless women in thongs while "working" in a kitchen with a big bowl of bacon on the counter that I could eat by the handful. Topless grown-up Vegas women and a bowl of bacon beat the seventy-two virgin houris vaguely and falsely promised to religious murderers hands down, even without the lap dance. I got strippers and bacon; the murderers just died.

Jet was teaching me cartoon mega SAD cooking, and that really started my journey toward health. Jet taught me how to take a beautiful, thick, deeply marbled (fat) steak, soak it in olive oil (fat), and then thickly coat it in a mixture of brown sugar (sugar), kosher salt (salt), and pepper (how the fuck did that get in there?), make a nice crust in a superhot pan (with added oil), and do the real cooking in an oven. This allowed me to cook steaks outdoors for a few hundred people at a medieval-themed restaurant in Jersey on TV, while making jokes, without measuring or timing anything. Guy Fieri said with professional TV hyperbole that my steak was the best he'd ever had. Jet helped me represent Vegas.

One of the things Jet taught me was to taste everything. He forbade me from putting any ingredient into a dish without tasting it. This meant I was tasting fish paste right out of the tube. It meant I was eating butter and kosher salt. Jet wanted me seeing, tasting, smelling, and even feeling every individual element as it went in. Neither of us knew it then, but Jet was getting me ready to really understand CrayRay when he taught me that the SAD was SOS. The TV style of cooking that Jet taught me (not Jet's real cooking style) made me understand that our American diets had so inured us to salt, oil, and sugar that it seemed no one could ever be busted for things being too sweet, fat, or salty. You could put in too much onion and lose a round, but two sticks of butter per serving were fine. I made classic Buffalo chicken wings, and that was just soaking fatty chicken wings in a vat of butter and then deep-frying them after covering them with something that would absorb the frying oil. Oh, and a blue cheese dip that was just fat and salt. Jet had me taste every single ingredient before it went in. I wasn't only seeing the sausage being made, I was tasting the offal as I made it myself. For weeks, with TV cameras all around me, I just dumped salt, sugar, and fat into bowls, heated it up, and served it with a story.

All the food I cooked was good. Jet did just what he promised to do. I cooked food that tasted great. Even with the very heavy leitmotifs of salt, sugar, and fat, there were subtlety and surprises. It was food that made the diner want more. The first bite knocked the judges on their asses—and after a few thousand bites, it could literally kill any of us. When CrayRay stripped me down to potatoes, when he stripped me of my American TV food tolerances, when he took away the fat, sugar, and salt and allowed me to taste something else, it was amazing. Just amazing. And it was Jet Tila, months before, who helped me understand what I would be giving up.

If you're lucky enough to go to one of Jet's restaurants, and even luckier to have Jet himself cook for you, don't expect Penn Jillette TV butter steaks. Jet cooks gourmet food with all the flavors. He's a fine "Rare and Appropriate" chef. And if you tell Jet that you want no animal products or refined grains and extremely low salt, sugar, and oil, Jet will make you a meal that you'll remember the rest of your life. Jet knows food. Jet and his family are also thin and healthy. He has a good relationship with food. He knows it well, but he sure taught me to cook unhealthy American TV food when I asked him to.

I got to the finale on *Rachael vs. Guy*. On the way there I cooked Thai chicken, Disco Fries, hot dogs, chicken wings, chocolate bread pudding, and spicy dark chocolate sauce with pink rock salt over doughnuts, and I finished in the finale with something I claimed I made up on the spot and also claimed had been my favorite for years (I wanted to give them choices in editing): Halibut Casino. I came in a very close second to Herschel Walker, who has been cooking all his life and owns a couple of restaurants. He made his grandma's fried chicken, and it was great. On reality shows, I don't win. I don't win because I don't know what I'm doing and I'm not the best (or because I accurately report that Trump's hair looks like cotton candy made of piss). But I have a blast muddling through these shows, and I put asses in the Penn & Teller Theater seats. That's the real game.

While I'm learning to do things on TV, I also learn things in life, and learning to cook with Jet Tila really taught me that I wanted something other than fat, sugar, and salt in my diet, and that might have been part of saving my life.

When Jet and I get together now, we eat wonderfully healthy gourmet food, but if some topless women want to invite us over to share a big bowl of bacon . . . I'm not sure we'll say no.

SALT—MORE PROOF THAT THERE'S NO GOD

More salt in my food equals more salt in my blood equals more water flowing to that salt in my blood equals more volume in my blood equals more pressure equals my ass shuffling off this mortal coil even sooner. It might actually be close to being that simple. Salt brings me real, provable pleasure, and it'll kill me if I let it. QED: we live in a godless universe full of pain. (If you need more proof, remember the difference in orgasm time between men and women.)

Salt causes volatile organics to be released from our food. So now you want to know what "volatile organics" means, but I don't know, either. I do know what they smell like, though: tasty goodness. And smell is a big component of taste (remember that stupid jive about eating a potato while smelling an apple, or, you know, oral sex). Salt also directly binds with our taste receptors and enhances flavor. When chefs say food needs salt to "bring out the flavor," they aren't talking about an illusion. These are real, physical effects. Salt makes everything taste better. It really does. Why? Why? Why?

"Salt" is another bullshit word like "protein," "carbohydrate," and "fat." Salt is just the product of an acid plus a base. It's what we think of as salt when the acid is hydrochloric acid (HCl) and the base is sodium hydroxide (NaOH). Caustic; scary.

$$HCl + NaOH = NaCl + HOH$$

The acid and base molecules get a little slutty, do a little swinging in the gated community that is chemistry, and swap atoms to form salt and water (HOH = H_2O). Intimate molecule swapping, as with humans, leads to some foam. The sexy fizz of baking soda (base) and vinegar (acid) forms a salt.

The problem is not salt in general but that very specific sodium ion Na itself, and the salt we love is salt with sodium. When NaCl hits H_2O, it turns into free Na and Cl floating around my body and fucking my shit. Magnesium or potassium salt are kind of close, but not close enough. We try to use these as "salt substitutes" to try to cheat our taste buds and avoid excess sodium, but they suck. Bummer.

Everything needs sodium to stay alive. Na is critical for all cell activity. For zillions of years it was really rare, and then we found shit-tons of it or got it out of the ocean or something, but we'd already evolved into salt-craving, salt-hoarding machines just to get our hands on some Na. As far as I know (there's a phrase that negates absolutely anything I write after it), pretty much no one dies from too little salt. I'm trying for none, and I'm still getting too much.

To colonize the rest of the planet, North American Europeans needed salt. We needed to preserve food. Genocide couldn't wait for refrigeration. We needed salt to preserve our food. Salty food was way healthier than spoiled or no food. Salt keeps bacteria from growing. Now with refrigeration and plenty of food, we don't need ham and pickles. We don't need bacon. We still love it, but what fucks bacteria also fucks our tissues and overloads our circulatory system.

American doctors used to say that a normal top blood pressure number was a patient's age plus 100. Yes, that was normal, but only because we were all salting our fat asses to death. For 90 percent of human history, we got less than a quarter teaspoon of salt per day. Now we get that much in one kernel of tasty popcorn. Down in the Amazon (the jungle, not Bezos's farm) there's a group of people called the Yanomami (when you write your anti-salt hip-hop anthem, I bet you'll be rhyming that with "hot pastrami"). The Yanomami eat a diet with almost no salt. No added salt. No animal products. Nothing refined. And their blood pressure doesn't get higher as they get older—not a bit. They have zero cases of high blood pressure. Meanwhile, in the USA you can kind of say that salt kills about 400,000 people a day. Salt kills more people than traffic accidents and bears put together. And bears are really mean and scary. Salt is worse than tobacco. I've been converted, so don't fuck with me.

But taste is habit (maybe there *is* a god . . . nah). At least that was true for me. I loved salt more than anyone I knew. I would add table salt to Mexican-restaurant tortilla chips and movie theater popcorn. I'd cook my eggs in bacon grease. I loved it. I couldn't get enough.

But salt was killing me. Not fat—salt. My goal with my CrayRay/Fuhrburger diet was to get rid of salt and fix my blood pressure; getting thinner so my cock looked bigger was just a side effect. So I cut out salt. It took a while, but I began to be able to taste small amounts again. After a few months of CrayRay, I could taste and enjoy the natural salt in vegetables. I now enjoy salt in much lower doses, so maybe I won't die as soon.

If god really so loved the world, he wouldn't have given us his only begotten son to torture and kill, he would have just made salt healthful. Seems easier, at least emotionally, right? And that's a gift we could really enjoy.

HALF-FASTS

Like a teenager, I keep a journal. Every morning I get up and write for about ten minutes about my day. More entries start with "I got up" than not. This is not creative writing, but I've been doing it since August 10, 1987. In my very first entry I wrote about how I've always wanted to keep a journal, but it's a little late because most of the stuff that's going to happen to me has already happened, so there's not much left. I guess I figured I was thirty-three years old and it was about time to be crucified. By now I've been keeping a journal for almost half my life, and it seems that a lot more shit ended up happening. With the help of my new diet, maybe I've got another thirty years; who knows?

My journal helps me forget stuff. Before I kept a journal, I would spend each day with conversations and ideas from the previous day swirling around in my head. For the past twenty-eight years, I've written my five to fifteen hundred words every morning and then forgotten about that day for a year, until I read that day's entry again. When I had been doing my diary for a year, I started reading what

I'd written the year before. When I hit five years, I started reading the entries from five years previous and then those from one year before, and then I'd write about my previous day. Now every morning I get up (see, I like to chronicle that), do at least forty-five minutes (I have a forty-five-minute, exaggeratedly named "hourglass" on my desk that I use to measure) of writing—for example, on this book—and then I read my journal from twenty years ago, then ten years ago, then one year ago, and then I write what's happened in the past twenty-four hours. I find that reading the old entries every morning is a way to time travel, a way to shout to myself across time. Before I was married, if a girlfriend could stand me for a year, the journal came into play. If I read that the year before I was having the same argument with the same woman I was having that very day . . . it was time to do something about it. The journal focused some breakups. Now I mostly read my old journals and cry. I cry at the memories of those I love who are now dead. I cry with joy at every little thing I wrote when our children were babies. I cry with embarrassment that I willingly sat in a room with Donald Trump.

I woke up (see?) yesterday morning and read my journal from twenty years ago. According to my records, I woke up and left for rehearsal without having any breakfast. I was a prick to Teller. I treated him really badly, and not just Teller—I snapped at everyone. I called my girlfriend at the time, a wonderful actor in L.A. She had an important callback audition for a TV show and had to work on that, so she couldn't fly to Vegas to see me. Instead of dancing with joy at her success, I pouted like an asshole about her not coming to see me and sucked some of her joy away. That's enough evidence that I'm just a prick, but in the journal I blamed it on not eating. I vowed that I would buy some cereal and eat that every morning. The solution for 1995 Penn was not to be more loving and considerate, it was to have some oatmeal in the morning.

Twenty years later, I now have a wife to pout about and still (always and forever) treat Teller badly, but I no longer blame it on food. It used to be that if I skipped breakfast, I had a hard time. I had to find a snack right away. Without food, my patience disappeared, I was snappish, and I even got headaches. That no longer happens, and I don't know why. I never know why any fucking thing is happening. But I cut and pasted part of my journal into an e-mail to CrayRay and asked him. He wrote back to say that it was a good question and he had no idea.

CrayRay and Fuhrburger both write about how people on the SAD don't know what hunger is. They have little rules of thumb: if you're "hungry" for a specific food, it's not hunger, it's a craving. If your thoughts are fuzzy, if you're headachy, weak, and snappish, if you're lethargic, if your stomach is growling and feels empty, that's not hunger, either—that's craving. CrayRay taught me with two weeks of potatoes what hunger is. I feel real hunger in my throat, and it leads to focus and patience. CrayRay writes some just-so stories about how evolution keeps you clear and energetic to find food when you need it. Our almost ancestors who didn't have energy to find food when they were starving died, and didn't become our real ancestors. It makes sense in the way things that aren't really true often make sense. I don't know the truth, and neither does Ray, but things have changed for me.

When I got up the morning I went on *Jeopardy!* (it was *Celebrity Jeopardy!*, which is kind of like remedial *Jeopardy!*, but we won't mention that again, okay? I won, that's what matters.), I did not have breakfast. If I had been on the show a year earlier, breakfast would have been planned out the night before. I would have had oatmeal with brown sugar and a banana, orange juice, maybe some bacon, and, what the hell, a couple of eggs over easy. I would have wanted the focus that comes with a good solid breakfast. I would have wanted to do my best and win (like I did!). But it wasn't like that when I went on *Jeopardy!* less than a year ago (and won). I got up and didn't eat a thing. The *Jeopardy!* people had a full and lavish breakfast spread for us at the studio (a year ago I would have eaten a second breakfast there), and the other contestants (the losers) were chowing down. I ate nothing. I went on the air focused with an empty stomach and I won (*Jeopardy!*; I won *Jeopardy!*).

Now, before any important meetings, I make sure I don't eat. I don't snack. CrayRay pushed hard to keep the fed window small. Because I like to eat before my show ("So you don't have to be focused for your show, Penn?" "Shut up.") and I like to eat after my show, I have my before-show meal at about 5:30 and my last meal of the day a bit after midnight. So, while I was losing I had about a seven-hour fed window and went only seventeen hours without eating.

It seems that when my diet was really high-calorie shit, I had to eat all the time. Now that my diet is low-calorie, I don't have any problem not eating. Years ago, if I was going to supper a little late and we had to drive to the restaurant and park and meet people and be seated and order—meaning it would be a couple of hours before I ate—I needed to have a spoonful of peanut butter and some cheese to make sure I didn't get snappish in the car on the way. Now if we go to a restaurant that doesn't have any food that seems right for me, I just have water and coffee, and I feel great. I don't understand it at all. Maybe CrayRay, Fuhrburger, and the Klap are right: maybe there is something like fat/salt/sugar addiction. I don't know.

My buddy Jason is an amazing juggler. He is a new kind of juggler, which he pretty much created: a jock juggler. When I learned to juggle, it wasn't a jock thing. I learned to juggle long enough ago that it wasn't even a hippie-knit-dirty-yellow-hacky-sack thing. When I learned to juggle, it was a freak thing. It was circus and carnival. At least in my twelve-year-old mind, when I learned to juggle I was doing it to be in Bob Dylan's dreams. I got really good before college students started doing it. I wanted to be circus. That was my only way into showbiz. Jason Garfield is a jock. He's a bodybuilder. His body is perfect. He is seriously buff. He's not as crazy as CrayRay—he's not CrayJay—but he's a bit eccentric. Before he met CrayRay he would come live at our house for months, and our kitchen would fill with his magic bodybuilding potions. Jason went to those strip mall "health" stores and bought every powder they scammed out, put it in a blender with egg whites and eye of newt, and drank it down ten times a day. It sure looked like the shit was working. He would shave his whole body and oil himself down and look pretty great. Jason was kind enough that when my wife was pregnant and on strict bed rest and bored out of her soon-to-be-motherfucking mind, he would shave up, oil down, get himself fully erect, and send her nude pictures. He's a good buddy.

Just based on the way Jason looks, he wouldn't normally be a friend of mine, but when he wanted to start the World Juggling Federation, he saw me as the most famous juggler and wanted me to do commentary for his juggling competition show on ESPN-17, which airs only in the Philippines. His goal was to take juggling away from clowns and jokers like me and give it to jocks like him. He called it "sports juggling," and you can see how it's caught on. The WJF doesn't allow any costumes or funny props or jokes. There never was much entertainment in juggling, but Jason is working to crush the little bit that remains. Juggling is now buff guys in sweatpants doing technical routines, every throw of which is harder than I could ever do when I was at my peak, while judges take notes and I do commentary. No one watches. If all the jugglers did it shaved down, oiled up, naked, and with hard-ons, maybe my wife would watch . . . you know, if they didn't juggle.

Since Jason and I both juggled and were working together to destroy juggling, and since my wife had him living at our house, Jason and I became friends. There was a brief time when both CrayRay and Jason were at the house, and because CrayRay talks to everyone about diet and because Jason's useless and dangerous potions were all around the kitchen, Jason and CrayRay got to talking.

After a few hours of talking with CrayRay, Jason went on our diet. I had seen only fat fucks do it before, but now there was a buff, shaved, and oiled guy doing it. Jason was skeptical of it, but he gave it the obsessive juggler try (we have that in common). Jason was thrilled with the results and became a CrayRay convert and preacher. Since there is no money in juggling (unless, you know, you at least try to be entertaining), Jason supplements his income as a personal trainer. When I hit my target weight and it was time for me to build my arms back up a little, I asked Jason to help me with biceps and triceps exercises, and by working out for just ten minutes every other day, Jason gave me nice arms. Not nice enough to shave and oil up or to look in the mirror and get my own cock hard, but nice. Jason is also working with me on a nice, clean five-club juggle, which I've always wanted. Jason is a great coach.

With Jason's bodybuilding and his ripped-off CrayRay diet, his clients were losing fat, gaining muscle, and getting healthier faster than anyone else at the gym in Seattle where he works. This was giving Jason more clients and more data points. Just a few months after we introduced him to CrayRay, Jason had gathered a lot of real-world data points on this diet plan. Jason didn't bring his clients through the potato famine, but he did have them go whole plants and use CrayRay's fed window. I sat in when Jason was talking to some new clients, and he had them promise to go sixteen hours without food every day, and he told them when they hit sixteen hours to try to go a little longer. He told them to view the feeling in their stomachs not as hunger but as the burning of fat. He was adding a kind of poetry to CrayRay's work. I liked feeling what I used to feel as hunger in a different way. And I liked the "try to go a little longer." I started pulling out my phone when I finished eating my second meal of the day and hitting the stopwatch. I'd try to make it sixteen hours before my first meal of the next day. Most days I do seventeen or eighteen hours before my first meal, and I usually hit twenty-two to twenty-four hours of "hunger" once a week. I keep a record of my time; it's another obsessive goal to make staying healthy fun.

Dr. Michael Klaper is a skinny, healthy old hippie fuck. He lives in Hawaii, and his wife teaches yoga, dances, and probably plays the hammer dulcimer. The Klap seems to know everything about digestion, and he's a great speaker. He's wicked smart—you know, for a hippie—and I love him. He's been so helpful. I have my doctor in Vegas who is wonderful and I run everything by him, but I write to the Klap as a buddy and he gives me a slightly different POV. He gives me the hippie POV, which I like a lot more than I like to admit in public.

I'm not qualified to even touch on this in passing, but Dr. Klaper does a lot of stuff with serious fasting. He runs the clinic where CrayRay goes for his long-term, serious water fasts. "Water fast" means "nothing but water"—it doesn't mean going without water. The last fast that CrayRay did lasted twenty-one days, and he loved it. The Klap doesn't claim that fasting is a panacea, but it sure seems to help a lot. In many of his cases, fasting has helped bring really high blood pressure to healthy levels in a very short time, and then it seems to stay there. This isn't something anyone can do on his or her own. You have to be in a medical facility that constantly monitors you. It can get dangerous to fix blood pressure that quickly. When I brought my blood pressure down with diet and weight loss, there were some scary days when my doctor was pulling me off drugs really fast and my blood pressure went too low.

I have begged the Klap to let me do a weeklong or ten-day fast to take all the extra fat off and to finally get off the low doses of meds that I'm still on, and he says "No, no, no." If I were willing to go to his clinic and have docs around and be monitored all the time, he'd let me give it a try, but that would mean taking a few days off from work, and I never do that. I just never do that. And if I could find time to take off, I'd want to be with my family instead of in some hippie clinic. It looks like I won't get a chance to do a serious fast, but I want to.

So I invented "half-fasts"—catchy name. The Klap says that a twenty-four-hour fast once a week is always fine, and forty-eight hours is groovy, too. He says I can go up to seventy-two hours without being in a clinic, but he doesn't want me working or traveling during those hours, and I'm always working and traveling during every seventy-two-hour period.

My life now is all half-fasts. On average, I do six days a week of at least sixteen hours before my first meal. My average is a bit over seventeen hours. I try to make sure that I hit over twenty-two hours once a week. As I write this, it's been exactly one year to the day since I started the CrayRay program. I'm about two pounds over my target weight at this second. I spent some time at ten pounds over my target weight. That means I gained about a pound a month. I couldn't keep doing that or I'd be back to where I started in nine years, so I took it off again. Before Christmas, when our business is a little slow, my children get a school vacation and like to go see their grandfather in St. Thomas (what a great place to have a wonderful grandfather). For sentimental reasons I ate only potatoes on December 9. I wanted to mark the day that CrayRay saved my life with potatoes. CrayRay and the Klap both seem to think that eating only potatoes is damn close to fasting. I had a few days in the weeks coming up when I didn't have to travel and I didn't have shows. I did short fasts during that time to get a little bit below my original target weight and managed to get my blood pressure down a little more, but the truth is I wasn't that goal-oriented. I like not eating for a while. I enjoy the energy boost and the focus.

·I used to think that magician David Blaine was an asshole for spending all that time not eating in a box in London. I thought he was just celebrating torture. I still don't think there's any art or entertainment value in it (he'd be better off juggling), but now I'm a bit envious. I now associate not eating with a certain kind of euphoria. I look forward to my next half-fast. It's hard to imagine that I'll ever have time to get to a hippie clinic and do more than three days, but there's no doubt I have the desire.

Not eating used to mean I would be headachy, ornery, panicked, and lethargic. Now not eating means I'm jacked up, happy, and focused. I love it. But I'm still a prick to Teller; diet won't change that.

[Note: I have all my data on half-fast dates and times without eating, but there may be enough laundry lists in this book already. But I have them.]

THAT'S NOT FUNNY AND IT
DOESN'T TASTE GOOD

CrayRay, Dr. Klap, and Fuhrburger all like to use the word "addiction" for the SAD craving for fat, sugar, and salt. I hate that word. I
don't have any idea what it means. Does it mean a physical need for
something? Yet food, air, and water aren't addictions? Some say it's
when there's a physical desire for something, when you need some
substance or activity to feel normal. So alcohol, crack, heroin, video
games, sex, and Facebook are all called addictions. My guys add in
salt, sugar, and fat. Those sure are things that I desperately craved,
and then when I cut them way down the craving stopped, but addiction? We did a *Penn & Teller: Bullshit!* episode about Alcoholics
Anonymous. Sometimes on *Bullshit!* we were accused of purposely
using full-blown whack jobs to speak for the side we disagreed with.
On that particular show we had Gary Busey, and he never supported
Trump for president. We made the points that AA is a way of having
government-forced religion, and that even by their own figures AA
is no more effective than doing nothing. What really pissed us off,

though, was the part of their program that insists on telling the heroes who lick alcoholism that they are powerless. It seems to me that when you kick an "addiction," you should feel powerful. As we worked with the researchers on the show, we couldn't find a way to define addiction that really held up and made sense to us. We tried to do the whole show without really addressing that idea head-on. So when my gurus used the word addiction, I bristled. It's a bullshit cult word to me. I guess they knew what they meant, but I don't.

I certainly went through physical changes. During my potato weeks I had some cravings for the diet I used to eat, but for a month or two before I started potatoes, I had already cleaned up my diet a little bit. I wasn't eating only pizza and doughnuts. It seems the people who start potato time directly from bacon and doughnuts have a harder time sticking with it. The first time I tasted celery after my potato famine, I was amazed that fucking celery, which is just water wrapped in dental floss, had real taste; it was even salty. If the definition of addiction includes developing a tolerance, then the salt-sugar-fat thing is certainly addiction. When I did my "Rare and Appropriate" or was working with Bobby Flay and ate two bags of plain yellow Lay's potato chips, it was amazing how the salt just fried my mouth. It was really hard to eat. And the smell and taste of "spoiled" oil was sickening. Many years ago I either read or made up that Americans love their potato chips fried in oil that tasted a little spoiled, and I didn't really understand it, but after not eating for a while it was sickening. After just a few months off black-tar potato chips, I could understand the tolerance part of their definition of addiction.

CrayRay told me that I had probably never felt real hunger before—I had just felt craving. He was trying to explain to an addict that there's a difference between the way you need China white and the way you need air, even though it doesn't feel that way. You can't wean yourself off air, no matter what my distinguished colleague

David Blaine claims on *Oprah*. What I used to call "hunger" wasn't really needing food. It wasn't really hunger; it was more like craving. After CrayRay, I came up with a test for hunger: if it's real hunger, I feel it in my throat; if it's craving, I feel it in my head and stomach. Real hunger is for any food: a Yodel, an apple, flaxseed, or foie gras all seem just fine. Craving is for specific stuff like a Double Whopper with cheese, my way (no tomato and extra mayonnaise), or even just something salty or sweet. I care about hunger now, but I don't care about craving. But these days it's easy; I don't really get cravings anymore.

The "addiction" they talk about is the way I used to feel about sitcoms and pop music. When I was growing up, we had one TV in the house, and my mom, my dad, and I all watched it together. We watched situation comedies, and I loved them. Then, toward the end of high school I started getting all counterculture, and in 1972 *M*A*S*H* came on and everyone thought it was so hip and funny; and maybe just to rebel, I didn't think it was hip and funny. I watched a couple of episodes and didn't like it at all. My mom and dad didn't like it because it was too hip, and I didn't like it because it wasn't hip enough. I stopped watching TV. Before I had watched TV every evening with my mom and dad, but now I was out with friends, listening to music, talking, laughing, being pretentious, trying to get to concerts, and trying to get laid; TV fell away.

After a few months of not watching situation comedies, there would come an evening when I wanted to hang with my mom and dad, and I'd sit down to watch TV with them like we used to, and what the fuck? What the fucking fuck? Situation comedies just sucked. I had lost my tolerance for laugh tracks and characters who never changed. I was reading a lot of books at the time—Vonnegut and Camus and Sartre—and there were ideas there. I was listening to Dylan and Zappa, and there were ideas there. But not on situation comedies. This was back before we all became unstuck in time with DVR and Netflix, and the goal of every situation comedy was to get into syndication. In syndication, writers couldn't count on people watching episodes in order, so characters couldn't ever change enough to make any random episode you happened to watch too jarring. Yeah, characters were added and went away, and even died, but there were no real big emotional changes and no big plot—just big arc. It seemed empty to me after my heart-healthy books and music, the laugh tracks jarring and the close-ups that underlined every joke distracting.

When I'd been watching a series every week, the characters were like my friends. I cared about what happened to them. But coming in cold, they were actors wearing a lot of makeup and mugging for the camera, with the same vanilla sex jokes and winking fart references. The jones was gone; the blinders were off, and I saw situation comedies for the suck they were. Or maybe they weren't suck at all, maybe they were great, but they were an acquired taste, like blue cheese, sardines, and olives. You gotta learn to like that shit, and then learn to hate the addictive salt in it.

When *Seinfeld* was on, everyone was watching. Everyone talked about how clever and hip it was. I know Jerry a little bit, and I really like him and love his stand-up. I watched five minutes of his situation comedy and couldn't stand it. Everyone loved *The Simpsons*, and P&T were even on it twice and I couldn't be more proud, but I don't watch it. I know some of the people who created the show and some of the writers, and they're funny, smart, and good, but I'd lost my taste for the form.

Food is the same way. I loved bacon and doughnuts, and there just didn't seem to be anything that was too salty or too sweet for me. I was on board. I loved the laugh track and the obvious close-ups.

Food doesn't seem like a habit, but comedy doesn't seem like a habit, either. I could get myself back into watching situation comedies, but I just don't want to bother. Why? I get so much out of books and drama and hanging out with real friends. And I could get back into sugar, salt, and fat, but I just don't want to. Vegetables are books. They have so much more variety and craziness while also being more wholesome.

FINALLY EATING LIKE
A FUCKING HIPPIE

Listen, I ain't no fucking hippie. I'm not. Yeah, I know, I was a fifty-nine-year-old guy with an impotent little ponytail and a stupid little goatee. And I'm a peacenik. Right when the Twin Towers went down on September 11, 2001, my first thought was, "I hope we don't kill a lot of people." I also worried about freedom of speech. As I sat in silence with my friends in a Starbucks a couple of days later, without even the sound of airplanes flying into and out of Vegas, I said out of the blue, "There go our civil rights." A few days later, I called my hero, inspiration, and getting-to-be-friend George Carlin. I was talking to him about the tragedy. George's take was a little different. Carlin's take was always different: he wanted to title the TV special he made right after 9/11 something like *I Kinda Like It When a Lot of People Die*. The powers that be didn't let him, but that's George. That's where he can live. I couldn't get to that place, but when I told him my feelings, he ran to get his notebook (I think he was still a paper guy) and read to me from his entries from the day of the terrorist attack. He read out loud to me, "There go our civil rights."

Yup—I went all peacenik. During a tragedy everyone does what they always do, they just do it more: government people want more government. Spooks want more surveillance. Generals want more war. I got more peacenik, more libertarian, and way more atheist. Later that fall I did a benefit at Maxwell's, the punk club in Hoboken, New Jersey, for the ACLU. I've always been fascinated by musicians doing covers. When Bob Dylan covers Blind Willie McTell or Lou Reed does "Blue Christmas," there's a lot to learn. So I wanted to do covers in magic and comedy. Comedians and especially magicians steal all the fucking time, but they don't do covers. They rarely admit that they're doing their own versions of other people's material. So Teller and I are adding into our Vegas show a hunk of The Great Tomsoni & Co., an act performed by our friend and mentor Johnny Thompson—the act he did to open for Sinatra in the '60s. We're using Johnny's music, his tux, and even some of his old doves. Teller is playing Tomsoni, so he has to learn the hardest magic that's ever been done by a genius, and I'm playing drums—so, I'm learning what drummers do. The bar is lower. In a Vegas bird act, there are drum hits, and I'll be delivering those as Jonesy, our piano player, plays the score that Johnny arranged (yeah, Johnny is a genius; he's the most knowledgeable magician in the world, writes jazz arrangements, and plays bass harmonica. He eats fire, played with Jerry Murad's Harmonicats, and wrestled Gorgeous George. He hung with Lenny Bruce and Lord Buckley and had the most amazing comb-over in showbiz). The "& Co." was Johnny's wife, Pam, one of the funniest people to ever try to walk and chew gum at the same time on a Vegas stage. She will be teaching our show-woman, Georgie, to fill those high heels. We're lucky we'll have Johnny and Pam teaching us (and I'm doing what Ringo could do).

I like the idea of covers. At the 9/11 Maxwell's benefits, Paul Provenza and I did Bob and Ray's perfectly written bit "The Komodo Dragon." Another night, Gilbert Gottfried and I did Abbot & Costello's chestnut "Who's on First?" Paul and I were faithful and stuck to the scripts. Gilbert . . . wasn't and didn't. But I was doing benefits for the ACLU when our country had such a hard-on for war that it couldn't even think about dinner first.

I could never call myself a closeted atheist, but after I saw what faith-based action really looked like on American soil, I got even more out of the closet. Teller and I wanted to help out our old stomping grounds of Broadway in whatever small way we could, so we did a couple of weeks during that horrible terrorist autumn in *The Rocky Horror Show*. A big fat guy like myself wearing lipstick and dressing in fishnets was a personal "fuck you" from me to all the hung-up anti-sex Abrahamic religions.

If guys who fly airplanes into buildings think we're too decadent, it's time to dress in drag and suck off a guy. If someone is going to kill innocent people just to make me feel terror, I'm going to wear fishnets and dance. Fuck them in the neck.

I'm so much of a peacenik that I didn't even want war after the attack on 9/11. I listen to hippie music. I love drug music. I'm not necessarily stoned, but I'm beautiful. As a matter of fact, I'm not stoned at all. That's one place where I separate from hippies: I've never had a drink of alcohol or a hit of any recreational drug in my life. I know I point that out too much. I'm not bragging—it's nothing to brag about—I'm simply saying I don't do something. It's just sloth. But it's often part of whatever story I'm telling, and most people don't read more than one thing I write, right? It's like the Stooges. The genius Larry (if you take George Carlin, Johnny Thompson, Bob Dylan, Lou Reed, and Larry Fine, you've got everything good in the world, as far as I'm concerned), was so upset that all the Stooges shorts were played on TV one after the other. When the Stooges made the shorts, they would come out at a rate of maybe a couple per year. They were only in theaters, so people wouldn't ever see them back-to-back. So if they did a similar gag a couple years later, the audience would have forgotten it. Try to think of me not trying alcohol or drugs as being like Moses calling Lawrence "Porcupine" a few times. It's supposed to happen a few years apart.

As sober as I am, I sure like drug music. Lou Reed used to parade me as an example of someone who loved the Velvet Underground but never did drugs. I could listen to "Heroin" and not do it. I'm the guy who never did drugs but loves VU. I've never met the guy who has never done drugs but loves the Dead. I'm sure not that guy. But I like most hippie music. I listen to a lot of beatnik music, but the hippie music is definitely there. My playlist has some Blue Cheer and Moby Grape along with the Stravinsky, Debbie Harry, and Miles (add them to the above list of all that matters in the world).

The other place I separate from hippies is my embrace of non-recreational drugs. I got a hateful message on my computer the other day from a man who called me a "Big Pharmawhore." He then wrote another message correcting himself to "Big Pharma Whore." I guess he looked it up. Well, I don't like the sex-shaming words, but I wrote back to him, in kind, that I was more of a "Big Pharma Slut" because I've never gotten paid for giving my sweet, tight, fishnetted ass to Big Pharma. But as much as I happily and without compensation suck Big Pharma's cock, I sure want to get off my few remaining hypertension meds. I've always thought it was amazing that hippies would take drugs manufactured and distributed by a stranger but were so wary of drug companies. Now that I'm thinking about my health more, I'm starting to see the craziness of my previous position. I didn't want to take black market drugs once in a while for recreation, but I was willing to take a handful of really powerful blood pressure meds that were certainly not more beholden to market forces than the local drug dealer every single day. It's now pretty clear to me that habitual med use can be more dangerous than occasional recreational drug use. Now I want both my high moods and my low blood pressure to be achieved without drugs, but my children got every vaccine they could get. I don't think the anti-vac people are hippies; they're rich, stupid assholes, right?

Maybe I'm not uncomfortable with hippies at all. Maybe it's that area where hippies and liberals overlap that makes me bristle. I was doing a lot of political pundit shows when Sarah Palin was in the news all the time. I hated the way liberals attacked her. They always seemed to be trying to find new ways to call her a "bimbo" while pretending not to be sexist. Women in the public eye seem not only to have to be attractive but to be attractive in exactly the right way. Sarah Palin didn't dress like the Left wanted her to. She was really easy to impersonate, and people started quoting the sketches as though Palin herself had said that stupid shit. It sickened me. So, I decided I was going to go on TV and stick up for Palin. I would go through the things she had really said and written herself, and . . . there was nothing I could stick up for. Yes, she was misquoted a lot, but the real stuff was also stupid shit. I hated the way she was attacked, but I could find nothing good to say about her. I had to grab the anti-Palin and the anti-anti-Palin positions. Kind of like I was anti-Bush and then anti-Obama. The stuff that I really didn't like—killing people, taking away liberties, and giving money to rich people—Obama, Bush, and Clinton agreed on completely.

Fast food was like Sarah Palin. The nanny-state POV on sodas and Big Macs is sickening. All the finger-wagging bullshit made me order my Triple Whoppers with extra cheese and mayo and add salt to my fries. I should have just carried a salt lick around with me. When well-intentioned friends would cook healthy food, I'd stop at McDonald's on the way to the dinner party, just to be an asshole. I thought eating Kentucky Fried Chicken was fighting the Man, but now it's pretty clear to me that the Man wears a white suit and a Western bow tie.

I still know that "organic" is bullshit even if they call it compost. I don't consider myself vegan or anti-gluten, but . . . I'm vegan and I don't eat gluten. I'm beyond; brown rice and spinach seem a little junk-foodie to me.

I'm gonna put on some Dead.

Peace.

THE HEALING POWER OF PRAYER

Some of my religious friends ask me if, as an atheist, I have a fear that I'm wrong and that some god will punish me. Nope. Never. I have no fear of god at all. No nightmares, no cold sweats, not even a rare disquieting moment. I don't feel like I'm rebelling against or disobeying god. There is no god. God is no worry to me.

I watched my mother, father, and sister die, and I didn't cry out to god. I've been in pain and been scared shitless, yet I've never begged god to exist and save me. I know there are atheists in foxholes—there's a military group called that—but I'm too much of a peacenik and a coward and now pretty much too old to ever be tested like that myself.

But I think I pray. When I lie in bed at night with my eyes shut, waiting for my personality to relax out of the muscles in my face, inside my head, with no one to call me on my shit . . . I pray. My mom and dad told me to say my prayers before I fell asleep, and I got used to spending that time thinking about what I'd done wrong in the past, and about what I hoped for the future. I call it "Penn's

Guilt Roundup," but I think some of my religious friends would call it prayer. During my prayer I think of the stupid and unkind (most often those are the same) things that I've done and how I could try to do them better next time. I think in general terms about how I want to make things better for myself, my family, my friends, and the world. I think of my family members and wish and hope things for them. As I get ready to write this next part, I'm feeling a little guilty already. I feel like I'm about to betray a trust that I have with myself. I allow myself to hope and dream before sleep because it's private, because I'll never be called on it. Now I'm about to call myself on it. I will try to be honest, but please know that I'm being very selective. To tell you more is too personal, even for a TMI motherfucker like me.

I fantasize that I find the cure for AIDS, save a lot of lives, and win a Nobel Prize. Lately I imagine I do *the* genius interview for CNN that brings Trump down for good (that would win *all* the Nobel Prizes, right?). I think about talking a suicide bomber out of killing himself and many others and . . . getting all the credit for it. I think about what MILF I'd LtF at my children's schools and how that might go down (I get stuck in a loop with this one now and again). I think about projects I'm working on being very successful and how that would feel. I think about projects I've done that have failed, but by some miracle are discovered to really be works of genius that were just ahead of their time. I don't want to be disrespectful to those who believe prayer is more than hope and fantasy. There are good people who sincerely believe prayer information is shared with a magic, all-knowing power. They're wrong, but I do know that to them, what I do isn't exactly the same as what they do. But I do believe there is some overlap in what's happening in all our heads when we're consciously starting to dream.

As an adult, I've enjoyed making these private nighttime prayer sessions a little more realistic. I make them a little easier to imagine. I don't imagine winning the lottery, I imagine the Penn & Teller Theater being filled for every single show (I do know the fact that there *is* a Penn & Teller Theater has already used up more luck than winning the lottery ten times in a row).

I used to wish that I were magically thin and healthy, but over the past couple of decades I changed that wish to "I wish I desired only healthy foods, so health would follow without magic." It's still magical prayer thinking, but with the artistic self-fake-out that I'm not asking for too much. It's filling a theater that already exists. It's a little more likely than winning the Powerball without ever buying a ticket.

I got into bed just last night and was running through ways I could have answered Teller more politely when he asked about me changing a line in the show. I thought about how I should have been more supportive of a plan my wife had for our family. I thought about MILFs, and then my mind turned to my health. I thought about what I could hope for that would make me healthier, and I had an epiphany. One of my prayers had been answered. I now crave healthy foods. This is not the first prayer of mine to be answered; I have my wife and children. But the craving for healthy foods is not one I'd thought about every night. After praying for that for years, it took only a little over a year with my buddy CrayRay to make that prayer a reality. About the worst thing I still often long for is peanut butter, and that ain't bad. It's pretty rare nowadays for me to crave pizza, steak, burgers, or brownies.

I've gotta talk to CrayRay; I don't really need to win the lottery, but maybe he could set up something with the MILFs for tomorrow's pickup.

WE ATE LIKE IDIOTS. WE NEED TO DIET LIKE IDIOTS.

"We ate like idiots. We need to diet like idiots." My buddy Andy said that. I had so many friends who were just like me. We ate the SAD with a vengeance. We ate doughnuts, pizza, and cheeseburgers like starving monkeys in a Dumpster behind the Mall of America. Now, with CrayRay, a lot of us have fixed that. As I write this, this book isn't out yet (heavy, huh?), but people have heard us talking on *Penn's Sunday School* about how we eat and have seen little articles in the press here and there, and every night after our show, with just that little info out, people come up to me and brag about how they've lost a shit-ton of weight, in some way inspired by us. They take out their phones and show me pictures of the two of us standing together just a couple of years ago, both of us fat fucks, and they're eager to take another picture of us together, both of us no longer fat fucks. People really want to eat better.

I was trying to add up how much weight has been lost by just my close friends. Joe lost 150 pounds, Andy lost, like, 70, Goudeau is around there, too, Matt's over 100, Richard is about 40, Rich is, like, 60, Michael is at 30, Cyan and Shari did about 20 each, EZ did 20, Frank was over 50 I think, and Brian was about 50. Tim and Leslie did over 100 together, BJ was over 70, and there's a lot I'm forgetting. I bet just with close friends like that we've lost over a half ton. Goddamn. Keep exaggerating a little, and my close friends have lost the weight of a cow dressed as an elephant. So many of my friends have gotten on CrayRay's nutty bandwagon that we'll probably end up hitting a ton. I have so many friends who were dying from eating like idiots and now are living from dieting like idiots. We try to fight full-on orthorexia by doing our R&As now and again, but it is definitely a cult thing. We are the ex-smokers who can smell cigarette smoke in the breeze a football field away and have to run over and give the poor asshole advice about quitting. CrayRay's first rule of CrayRay—don't talk about CrayRay—has fallen way away.

Every couple of years Penn & Teller do a Florida mini-tour. We hit Orlando, Melbourne, West Palm, cities like that, and play a Hard Rock or two and a casino and regional theater. During the tour I get to see one of my oldest and dearest friends, Crazy Kramer (I guess that should be "Krazy Kramer"). Kramer was a dark horse for the title of lifelong friend. He is a superstar record producer, and I knew him first through his music. When we did our last Bacon and Doughnuts Party with my NoGodBand, Kramer was there to play a song or two with us. While the stage was being set up, we had a private moment in the corner; he took my guitar and played and sang his song "Nine Minus Seven Is Two" while looking into my eyes: "I have a friend in a nuthouse in Paris / Strapped to his bed all alone / Pack up your troubles and sail away / Yankee, it's time to go home . . . I wish my father could see me now / See what a guitar can do." The combination of pure art and longtime love would have killed a lesser man. I'm proud that I just sobbed. John Lennon singing "Revolution 1" in the room with me right now, with Hendrix adding a lead line, could not have moved me more.

As the years have gone on, our friendship has grown way beyond music. Kramer's art and his heart have merged with mine. We were 1980s New York City friends driving around at super speeds in his Jaguar, chasing models. He moved to Florida to help the Amazing Randi do his skeptic thing and then just stayed there. He still flies around the world to produce any young band that wants help to sound their best, and then the Yankee comes home to FLA and reads and fishes. Like me, Kramer is getting gray, and we both still have our impotent ponytails.

When we first met, Kramer was a pothead and I was starting to get fat. Now, Kramer is as drug free as me, and I'm nearly as skinny as he. Kramer is one of the few friends who loved me enough to point out that I was too fat and said he didn't want me to die because of it. I didn't listen, because Kramer is a hippie. Kramer thinks that if he even has a taste of steak, he'll die. I always made fun of the way Kramer ate. We all made fun of his hippie shit.

It's coming up on my birthday. My deadline on this book is right around my sixty-first birthday, March 5, 2016. In the twelve months since I went from loss to maintenance, there was one time when my weight was up as high as thirteen pounds above my target. I sure didn't like that, but I now know what to do. I can dial it right back down. Right now I'm a couple of pounds under my target, and I like that. Last year on my birthday I felt great but I looked gaunt and sickly. My neck had more skin hanging off it than a sixty-year-old man should have. My face has since filled back out and my neck has tightened up. CrayRay's low-calorie, no-exercise program left me weak, but this year I have a different kind of muscle on my arms than I've ever had before. I have real, useful muscle now. Every week I do these super slo-mo push-ups and some weightlifting exercises that Jason Garfield

got me doing, and I now have the arms I want. They aren't as big as
they once were, but the muscle is defined, and I'm much stronger. I
do that torturous slo-mo stuff every Monday for eight minutes and
then take a week to recover, and by the next Monday I'm stronger.
Add in my *New York Times* app-driven seven-minute workouts, and
my formal exercise totals twenty-nine minutes a week. CrayRay says
the opposite of sedentary is not exercise but rather active. I'm active.
I play with my children and bound up the stairs, I practice juggling,
and I do the show with more energy and jumping around than ever
before. I live active, but I throw in that half hour of exercise a week
just to make Jason happy.

A month before this upcoming birthday I was sitting out on my
tiny hotel balcony in West Palm in the middle of the night watching
the rain fall into the ocean and talking to Kramer and his wife, Valerie. I love them both. My weight loss and health had Kramer choked
up with joy. We were old friends who might get a little older together
because of my changes in lifestyle. Kramer was pumping me for info.
He was telling me that every couple of weeks he has a piece of fish
and once a week he likes a nice big slice of bread with butter. Oh, and
pasta, he likes pasta now and again, too. Once in a while some yogurt.
He was confessing to me, the diet expert.

I was testifying to Kramer about how bread and butter and fish
and pasta and dairy and even his beloved honey were not good—they
were not part of the program. He was concerned. He wanted to learn
from me. Valerie and Kramer wanted to eat better, be healthier. After
they left I realized we were ass-backward. Kramer has been skinny and
healthy since he left high school and went to study music with some
Buddhist monks or some shit. He likes to carry on about a great kale
salad and a wonderful piece of cauliflower. When I used to take him
out to a steak house he'd have a piece of salmon and chatter about how
wonderful and rare for him it was. Kramer didn't really exercise, but

he'd walk every day to his favorite fishing spot, catch fish, and throw them back—he doesn't eat that shit—and then he'd walk home.

Kramer is an old fucking hippie. Kramer is the person we all made fun of. Now Kramer is the person we all want to be. I have all my R&As all planned out to enjoy a steak every month or so, and Kramer has a piece of fish when he feels like it, loves a little honey in his tea, and has some butter on his bread and a bowl of pasta now and again. This book is not written for Kramer. The last thing I want to do is thrust the other side of my pendulum crazy on Kramer. He's healthy, and his relationship with food is perfect. He doesn't need to think about this shit. He is, like Bob Dylan, playing guitar without tricks. He's just doing it.

I don't know if this book is written for you. I know for sure that my diet now is crazy. It's the way an idiot would diet. It's draconian and superstitious and, yeah, a little bit orthorexic. I know a lot about magical thinking, and this is it. I watch people eat turkey sandwiches backstage and I feel sorry for them; I think they're killing themselves. I watch people eat snacks and think they're crazy. I know that's wrong. Eating shouldn't be a thing. Eating is as natural as breathing; we just created a world where some of us were hyperventilating pure O_2 all the time.

I started this book by saying that you shouldn't take health advice from a Vegas magician. You shouldn't take diet advice from a fat fuck. And Kramer shouldn't take diet advice from a reformed fat fuck. I'm a zealot wearing a broccoli suicide vest to a Burger King. I know parts of this book are dead wrong. I just don't know what parts those are. I know I used to be sick all the time and felt like shit all the time, and now I'm healthy and feel wonderful all the time. It's not magical thinking to think that diet got me here, but I'm certainly no healthier than Kramer. I can't say I hope some of this book helped you, because I hope you don't need help. I hope you're healthy like Kramer. But if you are eating like a fucking idiot, maybe you need to diet like a fucking idiot. My way isn't the only way or the best way or the way I'll be doing it in a few years, but I don't want to go back to being a fat fuck. That was stupider than what I'm doing now. If you're a stupid fat fuck now, talk to your doctor, read CrayRay's book, and consider doing something about it. Then maybe after my show sometime we'll take a picture together. Two former fat fucks trying to be like an old hippie in Florida.

As another old hippie said, "Eat whole plants. Take walks."

"Arrows of neon and flashing marquees out on Main Street / Chicago, New York, Detroit, and it's all on the same street." Kramer and I both hate the fucking Dead.

But let's all try to make this long strange trip a little longer and stranger, okay, Krazy Kramer?

Thanks, Crazy Ray.

POTATO ANNIVERSARY

As the first anniversary of my potato famine approached, I dropped an e-mail message to a bunch of the other CroNuts asking if they wanted to do anything to commemorate the day. I wanted to celebrate by going through the whole famine again and got everyone all excited about it, but CrayRay wasn't thrilled with the idea. He reminded us that potatoes are not healthy eating. The idea behind the potato famine was to get me out of my bad eating habits so I could establish new ones, and it had done just that. Since it was just a psychological and physiological ploy to knock me out of my head for a couple of weeks, there was no reason to do it again. Although I was about ten pounds over the target weight I'd hit nine months ago, it wouldn't feel the same. I didn't need it, and since I was much thinner now, the weight wouldn't just fall off me. It would be less exciting. On top of all that, CrayRay was worried that I would write about it and talk about it and all his hard, complicated work would be seen as "the Potato Diet." That might get a little press and make us all some money, but it was bad science. I shouldn't go to just potatoes every December 9. CrayRay said that would be stupid and counterproductive.

So, at 11:55 p.m. on Tuesday, December 8, I had a few spoonfuls of peanut butter, and at 12:01 a.m. on Wednesday, December 9, I had a potato. I went against CrayRay. I'd gone rogue. I didn't have a plan, I was just fucking around. I wasn't going to do two weeks, but I wanted some sort of ritual. Last year potatoes were saving my life; this year it was just an unwanted performance-art love letter to CrayRay. I had a couple of potatoes during MovieNight that night with my buddies, but it was different this time, because no one noticed. None of my friends cared any longer if my eating looked weird. They couldn't bug me about it. It had worked, and I had earned my fuck-yous. Also, I was eating the potatoes with Tabasco, so it wasn't completely crazy.

I went to bed with a couple potatoes in my belly and got up the next morning and didn't eat. That also wasn't a big deal, because I had been going sixteen hours or more without eating on most days. EZ made me four bakers and a couple of sweet potatoes for supper.

I went in to do the show and had my low-calorie potato high. It felt great. I did a really fast, lean, fun, breezy show. Yeah, I got a little light-headed, but I still felt great. I had room service deliver me a bunch of potatoes after the show and ate two that night and saved the rest for the next day.

The next day, Thursday, was a travel day. We were going to play Harrah's Cherokee in North Carolina on Friday night. EZ grabbed me a few potatoes from the night before and added in a few sweet potatoes that she cooked up and a container of Tabasco, and off I went, eating potatoes to bring home the bacon.

I'm still using the CPAP. I still strap on my fat-fuck machine to sleep every night. It's a smart CPAP, so it measures how much I need it, and that keeps going down. I should get rid of it, too, but it gave me so much comfort when I was a fat fuck, and it's part of my sleeping ritual. It also means that TSA is even more of a pain in the ass, so I have my luggage shipped from hotel to hotel so I don't have to fight with the insolence of office (how did Shakespeare know about TSA?).

Because of the luggage being shipped, I just carried on a computer bag with my computer and my tablet and some plugs and wires. The potatoes wouldn't fit in the bag, so I had to carry a plastic bag with my snacks. Damn. I make fun of anyone in our crew who carries on a plastic bag from the sundry store. I had my fancy computer bag over one shoulder and a plastic bag full of potatoes and a Tupperware container full of Tabasco in my hand. I may be skinny, but I'm not classy.

The potatoes were wrapped in aluminum foil, the way the Rio prepared and served them, but I have since found out that can be dangerous. It's very rare, but in the anaerobic environment inside the cozy aluminum foil, the happy potato can fester killer botulism. You shouldn't store your potatoes in aluminum foil. You shouldn't even cook them in aluminum foil, because that's not a baked potato, it's a steamed potato. When one eats as many potatoes as I did for a while, people talk shit about them.

It was pretty much an all-day journey—two planes and a pretty long drive. I didn't eat a thing until suppertime, when we were changing planes, when I whipped out a sweet potato and ate it on the new plane after being seated. A cold sweet potato after I've lost my crazy SAD lust is like butterscotch pudding—creamy texture, and so sweet and pleasing. The guy across the aisle said to my manager, "I don't mean to be nosey, but is he eating a sweet potato?" The long-suffering Glenn affirmed his suspicion. I guess you saw that in the tabloids. When I got to the hotel I had another couple of potatoes with much too much Tabasco and slept great.

The shows we do on the road contain different material from our

Vegas show. A lot of the same people who see us in Vegas see us near their hometowns, too; we can only fit so much shit on the truck, and we like to change things up, so there's a different set list on the road and different bits to remember. Lots of different words I'm supposed to say, and a different order to say them in. I didn't want to be light-headed for a road show. I asked CrayRay about it, and he said that since he was against me doing just potatoes again anyway, he was okay with me breaking the potatoes that I shouldn't be doing anyway. The chef at Harrah's had taken the challenge laid down in our back-stage rider and made me a great meal. Broccoli, zucchini, black beans, brown rice, and a bunch of beautiful acorn squash baked just right. I chowed down and chased it with a couple pears. As usual, the first pear was great, and the second pear fucked me.

Zeke, my buddy and one of our Directors of Covert Activities, and I are obsessed with how pears fuck us, so we ran some scientific tests. I went to the fruit tray and grabbed a pear. It was sweet and juicy with a pleasing texture. This is how they fuck you: with this pear in my mind, I'm supposed to say, "I love pears, I'm going to eat them all the time," and then with pleasant anticipation grab my next pear—and it's sour or dry or mealy or rotten, and all the pears laugh at me. Fuckers. We tried to outsmart the pears. I grabbed a second one and, right before I bit into it, I ran over and gave it to Zeke. He tried it and it was perfect, juicy and sweet, its flesh supple, with just the right amount of give. He thought that maybe the problem was that taste buds change in reaction to the first pear, so he cut off a piece of his and gave it to me. It was delicious. It wasn't me; it was the pear itself. My mouth was fine. So I grabbed another pear and took a bite. Fucker! I've had worse pears, but it sure wasn't as good as the first one. It was a little sour, not as juicy, and the texture was a little funky. I grabbed another pear for Zeke . . . same thing for him. Yup—the pears had fucked us, so it wasn't our reaction to the pears. We didn't change; we had proved that. And it wasn't faulty memory between pears, because these were really close together in time. The pears were changing, and they were changing based on who was going to eat that particular pear. Amazing. How do pears know how to fuck a fellow? Zeke and I figured it was Schrödinger's pear. When someone picks up the pear it is neither good nor bad, or, more precisely, it is both good and bad at the same time. Juicy, dry, sweet, sour, ripe, green, rotten, mealy, and firm all exist together, superimposed on one another. It's a wave pear and a particle pear at the same time. Fuckers go quantum just to fuck our asses. So, I hit the stage in the Event Center at Harrah's Cherokee with an unsatisfying pear as my final food feeling. Fucker.

After the show I had some food-court pineapple and grapefruit. On the rare times that pineapple fucks you, it warns you: it looks a little brown or it's hard to the fork. Pineapple is the reliable booty call of fruit. Why go with that capricious, scheming, moody pear?

I had a couple of potatoes with way, way, way too much hot sauce in my room, and then an orange and some grapes to soothe the burning. I think while the pineapple was doing me a solid, the Dunkin' Donuts woman gave me caffeine in my "decaffeinated" coffee so I didn't sleep. I was up at 4:00 a.m. and had a pleasing apple from the fruit basket—let the pear cry itself to sleep.

The next day I flew home with a couple of Harrah's potatoes out of the foil and squeezed into my computer bag and ate the two potatoes on the plane. My Tabasco was in a regular bottle, so I could use it without stinking up the plane.

I got home, saw my family, and watched a couple of movies, and then I realized that I was hungry and what I was craving was fresh fruit. I didn't feel like potatoes, but I also didn't feel like a cheeseburger or a slice of pizza. A year later, and CrayRay's plan had worked. I've come a long way. I had some cherries, some blueberries with cocoa, and a handful of shelled pistachios. When I weighed myself, I was at 228.7. I'd lost most of the weight that I'd gained in nine months in just four days.

My little love letter to CrayRay was 6.2 pounds of fat gone in four days.

DEAR PENN

The groovy cats and kitties at Withings have invited me to write now and again about my "weight loss journey" (that phrase was in their e-mail). Their first suggestion was that I write a letter to myself ten years ago today: December 2, 2005, when my weight was way over three hundred pounds (I don't have the exact number because I didn't have my Withings scale then, and I didn't weigh myself very often, for obvious reasons—but it was about a hundred pounds more than I weigh now). December 2, 2005, is nine years, one month, and two days before I went into the hospital with blood pressure higher than UK voltage. Nine years, one month, and two days before my doctor suggested that I get a "stomach sleeve" to control my weight (I didn't do that; I got a scale instead).

Here's that letter.

December 2, 2015
Las Vegas, NV

Dear Penn,

You're wicked fat. People think they're being kind by not telling
you that. But even if they did tell you that, you're strong enough to
not be swayed by peer pressure. You're strong enough to not be swayed
by vanity. You're strong enough to not be swayed by the advice of
your doctor. You're strong enough to not be swayed by the fact that
you take a handful of pills every morning and night to keep your
blood pressure where it is: a red ——— hair from stroking out.

Our hero, Bob Dylan, sang, "To live outside the law, you must
be honest," and you pride yourself on having the strength to do that.
The New York Times *and the government tell you to take better*
care of yourself, and you eat a few Krispy Kreme doughnuts and feel
like you're sticking it to the Man. You aren't. I can tell you what no
one else dares to tell you: you are exactly like everyone else. You are
not honest; you are living well inside *the law, and you're doing that*
by lying to yourself.

You want to really live outside the law? Get healthy. Your
beautiful daughter, Moxie, just turned six months old. You found
out today that your next baby, who's going to be born May 22,
2006, will be a boy. You'll name him Zolten. Start telling people
now that it means "king" in Hungarian, so you're naming him after
Elvis, because you won't think of that joke on your own until he's
three months old.

You're a way-old dad. You were fifty when Mox was born, and
your life expectancy at your present weight is about another fifteen
years. Remember how you couldn't stop crying for a full year after
your dad died? You were forty-five then. How do you think Mox and

Z are going to deal with you dropping dead of fat when they're just teenagers, you selfish prick?

I've got an idea—why don't you grow some gonads and stop eating SAD (Standard American Diet)? Why don't you live outside the law and care more about your family than you care about hype? You didn't listen to the Eagles, you listened to Sun Ra. You didn't watch Seinfeld, *you read Nicholson Baker. You didn't drink beer, you learned to juggle. How come you eat like everyone else?*

I'm sorry, Penn, but you're going to eat like a hippie. You're going to be mostly vegan (but unethical vegan—no ideology, just health). You're going to stay away from refined grains, salt, oil, and sugar. You're going to just eat whole plants. The hippies were wrong about the Grateful Dead and socialism, but they were right about love and diet. You're a fifty-year-old man with a ponytail; you can be seen eating cruciferous vegetables.

Here's something you'll like: at first, weight loss is really hard. You need to take off in a few months what you put on in a few decades. Enjoy the difficulty. Everything you love in life, everything you're proud of, you had to work for. That's why you're proud of it. Don't believe the hype that there are easy ways to get healthy. Live outside the law. Be honest. It's easy once you get there, but it's difficult to start. You're bucking the whole system. The law says make things easy—so do things that are hard! Everything you love was hard to do: juggling, playing bebop jazz on upright bass, catching a bullet in your teeth, working with Teller, being married, raising children—even reading Moby-Dick *was hard. All the things that make life worth living take work. Don't believe the hype. Don't go on any diet that's easy and makes only small changes. Penn, please go crazy. Obsess. Change. Have fun.*

Live outside the law—and live there for a long time!

Oh, and by the way, on November 24, 2008, buy all the shares *you can of AssWhole Foods at $4.01 and sell them on November 29, 2013, at $64.95; in ten years, you'll be wicked thin, wicked healthy, and wicked rich.*

With love to your fat ass,
Penn Jillette

WITHINGS BLOOD PRESSURE CUFF—HAPPY VALENTINE'S DAY

I was in high school the first time I slept with my girlfriend. I'm not using a euphemism there. We had already done everything we could do sexually (at least, everything we could think of ourselves; this was before the Internet). We'd done it all outdoors, in cars, at school, even in bed, but we'd never slept together—maybe we'd dozed off for a moment for a nice little nap, but we'd never really fallen asleep for the night. Somehow, we were able to justify a weird trip on a houseboat together to our parents. They questioned our motives, and we were offended that they didn't trust us. In the end, we got to be alone on a houseboat and sleep together, a new level of intimacy for us. (What could this possibly have to do with Withings? They asked me to write "something sexy" about their blood pressure cuff for Valentine's Day. Watch me work.)

I learned a lot on the houseboat that night. I learned that even without the Internet there were some other sex things we could think of. I learned that actually sleeping together could be as intimate as sex.

I learned that when you've slept alone for seventeen years, waking up with a moving human being on your chest is really scary—like, heart-pounding, screaming, WTF-get-this-strange-living-thing-off-of-me scary. I learned that when a high school girl is sleeping on your chest and you wake up terrified and scream at her and throw her off of you and out of bed . . . it takes a long time for her to forgive you, find it funny, calm down, relax, and get back to REMing with you.

I also got to be in the same room with her when she brushed her teeth in the morning. A young woman brushing her teeth topless on a houseboat rates its own Internet subscription site, and I sure hope that site doesn't clone credit cards and sell them to China. I also learned that I brush my teeth really funny. There are no Internet sites for naked, geeky, too-tall, goofy young hippie men brushing their teeth. Supply and demand, I guess.

Her tooth brushing was sexy not only because of biology, physics, and standing waves but also because it was intimate. It was another level of sharing. Intimate to the nth degree.

I'm sixty years old now. I've watched a lot of women brush their teeth (even before my membership to that site—are you *sure* my credit card is okay?). What intimacy have I not shared? The most important number in health: my blood pressure. For a guy like me, who had blood pressure like the voltage from a British electrical outlet, there is no more important number. When I was losing my century of pounds last year, the Withings blood pressure cuff saved my life. I could not have lost that weight and got off of most of my BP drugs without it. There's no exaggeration there. The speed with which I lost the weight could have turned those lifesaving drugs into poisons on a daily basis. I didn't have time to go to the doctor every day to use his sphygmo-manometer, and I couldn't trust myself to call him and report ac-curately every time I took a reading. I would have called him every couple of days, and that wouldn't have been safe. The Withings cuff automatically sent my reading to him the instant it was recorded and allowed him to adjust my meds accordingly. My stupid-fast weight loss was safe and healthy because of Withings.

I'm going to call my wife in now to watch me take my blood pressure topless here in front of my computer. That's intimate and life affirming, right? Biceps are sexy. The cuff is kinda sorta like a little bit of bondage, right? Sitting still and relaxed after meditation, with your biceps in bondage, is sexy. What is sexier and more life affirming than taking one's blood pressure with a Withings cuff? I want to share that with my wife for Valentine's Day. What's sexier than that?

Oh yeah—a woman brushing her teeth topless. I have to get back to my site. My credit card really will be okay, right?

Oh, and for those of you who are wondering: 143/77 with a pulse of 61, right after writing this and checking out those sites and worrying about China having my credit card number. And now I've been intimate with you. Sexy.

LETTER TO THE *GLOBE* AFTER THEIR LYING ARTICLE ABOUT MY WEIGHT LOSS

Dear Ms. Allison,

Last week I ran to my mailbox, opened my newest issue of the Globe, *and was thrilled to see your byline on an article detailing how my recent weight loss was a "dirty trick" on my fans. It must be a trick, because it sure couldn't be willpower and knowledge. Do you reckon that since I am a Las Vegas magician, everything I accomplish must be done with smoke, mirrors, palming, false shuffles, and elective medical procedures? That's a common layperson misconception.*

But, Ms. Allison, you are so much more than a layperson. You have expertise. You are a health reporter for the Globe, *"a weekly tabloid focused on celebrity news, TV, music, entertainment, politics, culture, and true crime." That's a little like being the reality show fashion reporter for the* New England Journal of Medicine. *You may have some firsthand knowledge about my situation. I struggle*

*with lying in my job while still trying to be truthful in my life.
Know what I mean? I state onstage that I'm going to vanish an
elephant, and I don't—it's just a lie, or a "fib," as you call it. It's
just a trick. That's showbiz—I know it's not true when I say it, like
maybe some people know something's not true when they write it.*

*My recent weight loss was not a trick. It was my life. I was
in the hospital with some pretty serious hypertension issues. I was
scared. It seemed that improving my diet and taking off some pounds
might just give me a little more time and, more important, a little
more quality time with my young children. One of my doctors did
suggest a stomach sleeve, and it might have come to that, but diet
and willpower seem to have done the trick, so to speak.*

*Your reporting was secondhand, and the information you got
wasn't exactly accurate. In eleven weeks I lost seventy-four and a half
pounds. That's pretty intense weight loss, but it's not one hundred
five pounds in fourteen weeks. Adding some time to the top, I lost
90.6 pounds in 125 days. The 105 figure comes with adding a few
additional weeks on top of that. Before I started the really intense
diet, I had already lost a bit over fifteen pounds in a more relaxed
way. Those are the real numbers.*

*I did not count calories on this diet, so I just guessed at those
figures when I was pushed. I did use an extreme diet—maybe in
your terms a "fad diet." I ate no animal products and no refined
grains, and I severely limited my intake of sugar, salt, and oil.
Although some willpower was required, my health improved so
dramatically that the inspiration was easy to hold on to.*

*I don't know why your "North Carolina weight loss specialist"
would think anyone would do this without the direct supervision of
a doctor, but I was under very close medical supervision. This was
not a magic trick. It was not a stunt. It was not done for vanity. It
was done for my health. I have not suggested that the general public*

*adopt my "fad diet," and haven't (yet) even reported the particulars.
I was asked direct questions by a journalist who noticed my weight
loss and actually talked to me about it. I answered her honestly. I
did not lie.*

*My medical team, who despite not being vetted as health
writers for a tabloid gossip magazine still seem competent, felt that
my health was in much more jeopardy from being obese than from
quickly losing all that weight. My sphygmomanometer and meds list
seem to support that opinion.*

*I'm having some fun with this letter, but I had a very serious
medical condition, and I worked on the solution deliberately and
after much thought and consultation. I'm feeling better now than
I can ever remember feeling. I have some pride in my success and
how I attained it. I was hurt to see my accomplishments dismissed
in print, to be called a liar, and to have my concern for other people
denied.*

*You were right to caution people not to undertake extreme
health changes frivolously, but you were wrong to question my
integrity, sincerity, and compassion for others.*

*Thanks for your time,
Two-thirds of the Penn
Jillette I used to be*

NO, REALLY, WHAT THE FUCK DO YOU EAT LIKE NORMALLY?

I've covered what the rules are for my diet. I bragged about how I got a fancy-ass chef to cook for my birthday. I've confessed my "Rare and Appropriates" where I go pig-nutty and gorge on bacon, doughnuts, corned beef, ice cream, pizza, and other shit. But what do I eat day-to-day? A healthy diet is all in the day-to-day; outliers in either direction don't matter.

Some asshole journalists seem to think that I was able to lose weight because I've got enough money. My weight loss, they presume, is too expensive for a regular Joe. Well, if that regular Joe is Joe Swam, it ain't true. Where I lost just over a hundred pounds, Joe lost one hundred fifty pounds, and he has some sort of civilian job at a supermarket or something. He started out as a fan and became a friend. Joe says, "There's no 'I' in 'team' and no 'eat' in 'entertainment.'" Joe is a happy CroNut who seems to get more entertainment from plants than he claims to. If you've got enough money to get fat, you've got enough money to get thin. I needed some doctor visits, because at the speed I was losing weight my doctor had to really watch my blood pressure. I bought a Withings Wi-Fi scale and BP cuff, and those were a couple hundred bucks, which is a bit of a jingle, but I didn't absolutely need them. I don't have a private chef. If anything, my food got cheaper by a lot, because I used to eat every day at a restaurant and now it's about once a month. Food at home is cheaper. I saved more money than others will because I spent more. I think most any American eating a SAD would save some money eating the way I do, and I'm not figuring in how expensive it is to be a fat fuck, with doctors' bills and sick days without work, I'm just talking food.

All that being said, my wife loves to cook, and she's eating the same food I am and she loves exploring the Fuhrbuger recipes and trying new things, so I do kind of have a private chef, and she's the best. But it's the same as she would do if she were cooking for herself—just more food. When my wife goes away for vacations (I don't take them), she leaves me with some stews and soups, but I can get by on things that even I can prepare. I could eat this diet pretty cheaply by myself.

I've been pretty good about not quoting Bob Dylan too much in this book, but Bob sang, "I can live on rice and beans." CrayRay isn't crazy about rice in the diet, but I like it. A meal for me, when my family is gone, is a big bag or two of triple-washed salad greens (that hippie kale kind) with some apple cider vinegar. How does that jingle compare to a Big Mac? Not too bad. I throw some brown rice in our fancy-ass rice cooker earlier in the day, and it's all ready for my supper. Target (that super-rich-guy store where you bump into Bill Gates all the time) has low-sodium Simply Balanced beans of all kinds in little cardboard boxes that you fold over and rip the top off of (my wife had to teach me, but I'm an idiot; you can figure it out yourself). I put the beans in a colander and rinse them off because I don't like the creepy, slimy bean blood all over them. I put a couple of boxes of those beans

in a bowl and spoon the hot brown rice on top. The beans are a buck
and a half a box, and rice is cheap, right? I sometimes just let the rice
heat up the beans, and sometimes I put them in the microwave for a
minute. I then put some Tabasco and some nutritional yeast on top,
and that's a meal for me. Salad, beans, and rice. Gotta be under six
bucks, right? And about ten minutes of preparation.

Because I do my half-fasts all the time, I have that salad/beans/
rice meal after at least sixteen hours and usually eighteen hours of
not eating. For dessert I always like to have some fruit. I'm too lazy
to cut up watermelon, but they sell it already cut up and in plastic; I
guess that's a rich-guy thing, so cut up your own fucking watermelon.
I sometimes eat two big containers of watermelon, and I love them.
My wife loves to peel oranges and grapefruits (or so she claims), but
they sell those already peeled, too. I like my fruit really cold, right out
of the fridge and ready to eat. A couple of plastic containers of watermelon, and we're still under ten bucks and fifteen minutes.

If I'm still hungry after all the salad, rice, beans, and fruit, I have
some raw, unsalted, nothing-added nuts. If I'm feeling fancy I'll have
pistachios; if I'm slumming I have peanuts (dry-roasted; raw doesn't
swing with peanuts). A handful of those bad boys will give you calories to spare. When I was losing weight, I *never* did fruit or nuts, but
for maintenance they're fine and I love them.

After the show, I might have some guacamole or hummus. Sometimes I have hippie peanut butter and then regret it because it's really
high-fat and high-calorie. After the show I almost always have fruit—
cantaloupe, kiwi, apples, peaches (not pears—they'll fuck you), or
berries. Ah, berries, let's talk berries.

The best idea I ever had was asking smart girls in my high school
class to fuck. Fucking smart girls was the best idea of my life. It gave
me hours of entertainment, my wife, my children, and everything I
live for. I should have gotten the Nobel Prize for that. My second-best

idea was hot-choco-berries. You are going to love me for this. This one is a little expensive, but worth it.

I take a big old colander and dump in a *lot* of berries. I mean a *lot*. Stupid lot. I use only blueberries and blackberries. I don't fuck with strawberries, because you have to cut the green shit out of them, and I don't trust raspberries, because they get moldy too fast. Now, blackberries and blueberries are expensive if you buy the bullshit "organic" AssWhole Foods ones, but Sam's Club has berries, too, and they're much cheaper (but they're a fancy private club where you might bump into the Koch brothers). Those little plastic containers hold a pint, and I'll do, like, four pints each of blackberries and blueberries. Sam's has bigger containers, too. That's a *lot* of fruit. I put the berries in the colander and rinse them off well (in case they've been near a Chipotle). I then dump them into a big stainless-steel bowl. I *love* big stainless-steel bowls for salad and fruit. The berries are cold and a little wet-reflected around the shiny bowl. On this chilly deliciousness I sprinkle (dump) a lot of cayenne pepper—I mean a lot of that dangerous orange/red (nature's warning sign) goodness. This gives it a real pop and keeps wimps out of my fucking berries. You sprinkle on as much cayenne as I do, and no one can fucking eat it. I choke and cough and love it. I shake the bowl around to get the spicy poison well distributed over the berries. When that's done, I take some Fuhrburger plain cocoa. This is real chocolate—no fat, no sugar, just brown and bitter. I put on way too much. I dump it in. This is fancy Fuhrburger cocoa powder, so it's not cheap, but it's certainly not as expensive as one dessert at TGI Fridays.

The taste is amazing. It's like a Mexican flourless chocolate cake. It has a lot of sweet from the berries, but it's still got that bitter, so bitter, as bitter as a shitty journalist writing about a rich Vegas magician's diet. The cayenne burns the shit out of your mouth, and the cool, gentle berries soothe you. The bitter makes you pucker until the berries lay their sweetness on your tongue. The texture is perfect, decadent and goofy. Eat them with a big soupspoon. Don't even attempt it with your fingers—that cayenne almost burned my jazz-bass calluses off my fingers. My habits and microbiome have changed; I don't crave doughnuts ever anymore, but I crave my hot-choco-berries all the time. They're so filling, and if you chase them with a small handful of peanuts, you won't be hungry for hours, and that sweet hot will make you sweat. Once I dumped handfuls of peanuts right in with the berries, and . . . well, it was so good, I could be back to three hundred pounds again in no time. I'm telling you, this is my second-best idea.

If I didn't have EZ for my wife, this is what I would eat all the time. I might try to throw some onions, mushrooms, carrots, and beets into my salads and some onions on the beans (I love onions), but I think I could get by on this. Add an R&A every couple of weeks, and I'd be swinging. Healthy and happy and, all things considered, probably cheaper than what you eat now.

If you're more ambitious and have a bit more time and money and like a bit more variety, my wife has taken a lot of the CrayRay and Fuhrburger ideas and run with them. Here are some of the foods she makes for us all the time.

EZ'S NOT-QUITE-EZ MEALS

PHONEY ISLAND HOT DOG

FOR THE HOT DOG:
2 cups cooked black beans
2 avocados
4 cloves chopped
⅓ cup fresh tomatoes, chopped
½ medium green bell pepper, seeded and chopped

1 jalapeño pepper, diced and seeded

3 green onions, chopped

⅓ cup chopped fresh cilantro

2 tablespoons fresh lime juice

1 teaspoon ground cumin

1 teaspoon chipotle chili powder

8 large romaine or Boston lettuce leaves

In a bowl, mash the beans, avocados, and garlic together with a fork until well blended. Add all ingredients except the lettuce and mix. Use your hands to form a "hot dog" and roll it into a lettuce leaf.

FOR THE SAUERKRAUT:

1 green cabbage, shredded

1 tsp caraway seeds

5 sprigs of fresh dill weed, minced

1½ cups cider vinegar

¼ tsp ground mustard

¼ cup of apple juice

⅓ cup of water (or more if you don't like it so tangy)

Put all ingredients into a medium pot and bring to a boil. Cover, reduce heat, and simmer for 25–40 minutes. If it starts to get dry, add some water. Remove from heat and let cool.

Add this sauerkraut to the hot dog and garnish with salt-free mustard.

CAPREZ

3 heirloom tomatoes

1 red onion

lots of fresh basil

balsamic vinegar

orange rind

Mrs. Dash seasoning

Slice the heirloom tomatoes and onions and alternate them on a plate. Chiffonade the basil and cover the tomatoes and onions with it.

Put the balsamic vinegar and orange rind into a medium pot and reduce to a glaze (15–20 minutes). Lightly drizzle glaze over everything on the plate, then sprinkle with Mrs. Dash.

TAFOOLIE

½ cup bulgur

1 cup boiling water

⅓ cup freshly squeezed lemon juice

2 cups cooked chickpeas

1 pound broccoli florets, finely chopped

4 scallions, thinly sliced

1 cup finely chopped parsley

½ red bell pepper, finely diced

¼ cup nutritional yeast

6 cloves garlic, minced or pressed

½ cup craisins

freshly ground black pepper

Boil the bulgur. In a separate bowl, combine the remaining ingredients and stir well to combine. Add the bulgur and combine thoroughly. Taste and adjust the seasonings by adding more lemon, garlic, or pepper if desired. Cover and let the flavors blend together in the refrigerator for about an hour.

Finally, here is what we eat the most. We have this at least once a week, and when we need to drop a few pounds we have this every day until we're back on track.

CORN-TOM STEW

1 can/box black beans, cannellini beans, or kidney beans, rinsed

1 can no-salt-added crushed tomatoes

1 can no-salt-added tomato sauce

2 cups butternut squash, cubed to bite size

8 cups low-sodium veggie broth

2 cups roasted corn

1 medium onion, chopped

3 stalks celery, chopped

6 cloves garlic, sliced

2 bay leaves

1 tsp thyme

1 tsp oregano

1 tsp paprika

Lay the corn out on a baking sheet and roast for about 20–30 minutes until golden or brown.

Sauté the celery, onion, and garlic in some of the veggie broth. Once they're softened, add the rest of the broth, the rinsed beans, butternut squash, tomatoes, tomato sauce, and all the herbs and spices (basically, everything else!). Let simmer for at least an hour. Thicken with tomato sauce, thin with broth. Add hot sauce and eat all day.

ACKNOWLEDGMENTS

Motherfucker, isn't Ray Cronise thanked enough in this book already? But you know, he kind of saved my life, so it doesn't hurt to thank him again.

Emily Zolten Jillette, my wife, known as EZ, made all the food I eat, and I guess she saved my life, too, but she'd already saved my life a zillion times before, so I'm kind of used to it.

Mox and Z, our children, watched a third of their dad go away and had to adjust to Daddy eating weird shit. They let me sniff their Doritos.

Dr. Joel Fuhrman gave our family recipes on which to build our new lifestyle. Dr. Michael Klaper is just an inspiration, a happy hippy genius who eats right and knows shit. Thanks to my personal Vegas doctors, who watched me get healthy, and took me quickly off my life-saving drugs before they became life-threatening drugs.

Jason Garfield is a great juggler and a piece of ass. He knows a lot about exercise. Once I hit target weight, he was really helpful in getting my strength and fitness back. Even if I were willing to work as hard as he does on exercise, I still couldn't look like him, so fuck it.

I need to thank all the "CroNuts," the groovy cats and kitties who went on this journey with me and gave me a lot of advice on what it felt like to people other than me. Michael Goudeau is a great friend, and he started this journey with me. I love Goudeau. Here are the others who have lost a shit-ton of weight with CrayRay and talked to me about it: Matt Donnelly, Joe Swam (he also gave me the Flinstones vitamin joke), Andy Lerner, Rich Ross, Richard Frankel, Emery Emery, Heather Henderson, Lana Strong, Dr. Brian Iriye, Frank Kassela, Cyan Banister, Shari Getz, James Messina, Mike Wilson, Kristy Pitchford, Tim Jenison, Leslie Jenison, Carr Hagerman, BJ Kramer, and Danny Greenspun.

Robbie Libbon has been my friend since we were teenagers. He works on the Penn & Teller Show, and he worked his ass off on this book. He knows grammar and logic and punctuation, and he also knows me; much of this book was Robbie understanding what I was trying to say and then putting it in my own words. It's a hard job, and he's great at it.

There's a lot of business that goes into making a book, and I want to thank all the people who do all the grown up stuff for Penn & Teller: Laura Foley, Steven Doctors, Kathleen "Burt" Boyette, Glenn Schwartz, Pete Golden and, of course, the long-suffering Glenn Alai, who is so much better at being me than I am.

The Simon & Schuster team: Ben Loehnen, Jonathan Karp, Larry Hughes; and my agent, Steve Fisher.

Always thanks to Teller. He's put up with Fat Penn, Skinny Penn, Becoming-Fat Penn, Becoming-Skinny Penn, and, well, me. He's my partner.

Oh, and remember, CrayRay and EZ saved my life.

ABOUT THE AUTHOR

PENN JILLETTE is a cultural phenomenon, both as a solo personality and as half of the world-famous Emmy Award–winning magic duo Penn & Teller. He has appeared on *Dancing with the Stars*, *Celebrity Apprentice*, *Modern Family*, *The Tonight Show with Jimmy Fallon*, and hosted the NBC game show *Identity*. He currently cohosts *Penn & Teller: Fool Us* on The CW, in addition to his legendary magic show, now in its fifteenth year at the Rio All-Suite Hotel & Casino.